Workbook for
The Nursing Assistant
Acute, Subacute, and Long-Term Care

Fourth Edition

JoLynn Pulliam, BSN, MS, RN
Nurse Administrator/Nurse Recruiter
Nursing Education Support
St. Mary Mercy Hospital, Livonia, Michigan

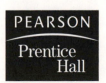

PEARSON

Prentice
Hall

Upper Saddle River, New Jersey 07458

NOTICE

Care has been taken to confirm the accuracy of information presented in this book. The authors, editors, and the publisher, however, cannot accept any responsibility for errors or ommissions or for consequences from application of the information in this book and make no warranty, express or implied, with respect to its contents.

The authors and publisher have exerted every effort to ensure that drug selections and dosages set forth in this text are in accord with current recommendations and practice at time of publication. However, in view of ongoing research, changes in government regulations, and the constant flow of information relating to drug therapy and drug reactions, the reader is urged to check the package inserts of all drugs for any change in indications of dosage and for added warnings and precautions. This is particularly important when the recommended agent is a new and/or infrequently employed drug.

Publisher: Julie Levin Alexander
Assistant to the Publisher: Regina Bruno
Editor-in-Chief: Maura Connor
Executive Editor: Barbara Krawiec
Assistant Editor: Sladjana Repic
Development Editor: Maureen Muncaster
Editorial Assistant: Christopher DiLeo
Director of Manufacturing & Production: Bruce Johnson
Managing Production Editor: Patrick Walsh
Production Liaison: Mary C. Treacy
Production Editor: Karen Ettinger, *The GTS Companies*/York, PA Campus
Manufacturing Manager: Ilene Sanford
Manufacturing Buyer: Pat Brown
Design Director: Cheryl Asherman
Senior Design Coordinator: Maria Guglielmo Walsh
Director of Marketing: Karen Allman
Executive Marketing Manager: Nicole Benson
Marketing Assistant: Patricia Linard
Marketing Coordinator: Michael Sirinides
Channel Marketing Manager: Rachele Strober
Composition: *The GTS Companies*/York, PA Campus
Cover Printer: Phoenix Color
Printer/Binder: Bind-Rite Graphics, Inc.

Pearson Education Ltd.
Pearson Education Singapore Pte. Ltd.
Pearson Education Canada, Ltd.
Pearson Education—Japan
Pearson Education Australia Pty. Limited

Pearson Education North Asia Ltd.
Pearson Educación de Mexico, S.A. de C.V.
Pearson Education Malaysia Pte. Ltd.
Pearson Education, Upper Saddle River, New Jersey

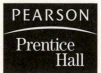

10 9 8 7 6 5 BRR 09 08
ISBN 0-13-119641-3

CONTENTS

Introduction

Training to become a nursing assistant is challenging and rewarding. This workbook will help you get the most out of your training program, whether you are preparing for a career in acute care or long-term care.

The workbook is designed to accompany your textbook, *The Nursing Assistant: Acute, Subacute, and Long-Term Care,* fourth edition. It is organized into the following sections:

- **Preparing for the Competency Evaluation.** This section provides guidelines that will help you prepare for the written and skills tests. Subjects include how to begin to prepare, how to study, how to answer multiple-choice questions, and how to develop test-taking strategies.

- **Skills Checklist.** This is a complete listing of all the procedures described in the student test. As you successfully demonstrate each skill, have your instructor initial and date the procedure listed.

- **Learning Activities.** At the beginning of each chapter in this section, you will find a MediaLink box. Just as in the main textbook, this box identifies for you all specific media resources and activities available for that chapter on the CD-ROM which is found in the main textbook and the Companion Website. The 24 chapters of Learning Activities are keyed to the 24 chapters in your textbook. Different types of activities help make sure you have understood what you have read in your textbook chapter. Many activities ask you to put yourself in the shoes of a nursing assistant and explain how you would handle real-life situations.

- **Quizzes.** The 24 chapter quizzes test your knowledge of the key concepts in the chapters. The multiple-choice format gives you an opportunity to practice the kinds of questions you will need to answer in your written test.

If you have difficulty answering any of the questions in this workbook, speak to your instructor. He or she will be able to offer guidelines for dealing with problems.

Preparing for the Competency Evaluation

Because nursing assistants work so closely with patients, the federal government has established guidelines and requirements for nursing assistants in different working situations. In fact, nursing assistants who work in long-term care facilities and many who work in acute care facilities must be certified. To get certified, you need to complete a state-approved training program. You must also take and pass a written test and a skills test. The tests, which are also referred to as a competency evaluation, determine whether you have the knowledge and skills to provide patients with safe care.

Beginning to Prepare for the Evaluation

How can you begin to prepare for the competency evaluation? First, you can pay close attention to your instructor during your training program. You will be taught the essential information and skills that you need to know. Don't be afraid to ask questions if you don't understand something. Your instructor's job is to help prepare you to be an effective nursing assistant.

Second, use your book to study. Read it carefully and completely. Use the step-by-step directions in the book to practice each procedure. Make sure that you can answer the review questions and perform the procedures in each chapter. Those questions and procedures deal with the key concepts and skills that will be tested.

Third, use this workbook to reinforce your knowledge. The learning activities and quizzes will help you to test your comprehension. If you can't complete a question or if your answer is incorrect, go back to your book and reread that section until you understand it completely. The skills checklists are designed to ensure that you have learned how to perform each procedure. You will need to be able to demonstrate some of those procedures to pass the skills test.

The following sections can also help you to prepare for the competency evaluation. You will learn how to study for the tests, how to answer multiple-choice questions, and how to prepare for test-taking. If at any time you feel that you need additional help, talk to your instructor.

Studying for the Tests

Studying is the key to performing well on the competency evaluation. Many people, however, do not know how to study effectively. In this section, you will learn how to organize your study time so that you'll get the most out of it.

First of all, you need to give yourself plenty of time to study. Set aside one, two, or three sessions a day for several weeks before the evaluation. It's always better to feel overprepared than underprepared.

Choose your periods of greatest energy for study sessions. If, for example, you're always tired in the evening, plan to study earlier in the day. People who work during the day might study first thing in the morning, during their lunch hour, or right after work.

Sessions should last from 45 minutes to 2 hours. Start by studying for 45 minutes to an hour at a time, and build up to 2 hours. If you start to lose your concentration or you feel very tired during a session, stop. You need to be mentally and physically alert for studying to be productive.

Study in a systematic manner. Don't hop around from subject to subject. Study all of one chapter before you move on to another.

Pick one day a week to review sections that you've already studied. This will help you retain the material. A friend, relative, or member of your training program can help you go over material or practice procedures.

Whenever you study, keep in mind that your attitude will affect how well you study and how well you do on the evaluation. At all times, relax and think positively. Being anxious or pessimistic won't help you accomplish anything. In fact, it may actually hurt you.

Answering Multiple-Choice Questions

The written test consists of multiple-choice questions. There are four possible answers to each question. You need to choose the *one best* answer to the question.

Here are some guidelines you can follow that will help you when you answer the questions:

- Read the question and all four of the answers carefully and completely before you select the *one best* answer.
- If you don't know the answer to a question, skip it and go on to the next question. You may remember later or get a clue from another question. Just be sure that you don't forget to go back to complete unanswered questions.
- When answering a question you're not sure of, eliminate answers that you're sure are wrong. Then choose one answer. If you don't answer the question, it will definitely be counted as wrong.
- Beware of answers that include words such as *always, never, all*, and *none*. They do not allow for exceptions.
- If you have time, go back over the test to make sure that you gave one answer for each question. Don't change answers unless you're sure they are incorrect. Your first reaction is usually correct.

Guidelines for Taking the Tests

Before you can take the tests, you must fill out an application form. Your instructor can help you obtain a form. When you send in your application form, you will also be required to pay a fee.

After your application form has been processed, you will be notified about the time and place of your tests. You will receive an admission card that you must bring to the tests.

The written test and skills test may be taken on different days, at different times, and in different places. Be sure that you know how to get to all testing sites and that you allow yourself plenty of travel time. If you're unsure, you may want to make a trial run a few days before the test.

Before the Tests. Test-taking success depends to a large extent on what you do during the 24-hour period before the test as well as on what you do during the test:

- After weeks of systematic studying, you shouldn't need to study the night before the test. In fact, you're better off relaxing and getting a good night's sleep.
- Eat a nutritious meal before the test. Protein foods, such as meat, milk, or eggs, and complex carbohydrates are your best bets because they'll help you stay alert.
- Dress comfortably but not too warmly. If you're too warm, you might get sleepy.
- Be on time but not too early. If you are late, you may not be permitted to take the test. If you have too much time, you may get nervous.
- Bring a form of photo identification, such as a driver's license, and another form of identification that has your signature on it.
- Bring your admission card and your Social Security number.
- Don't take any books or notes with you. You won't be allowed to take them with you into the testing room.

During the Tests. Listen carefully and follow all instructions. If there's something you don't understand, ask before the exam begins. Don't rush through the test—you will have plenty of time to complete it.

Taking the Skills Test

The skills test varies from state to state. You will be given a set amount of time to perform a specific number of procedures. You will be told which skills to perform when you arrive at the test site. A registered nurse will evaluate your performance.

The exam will be based on your skills, on how you treat the patients, and on your use of safety practices. These will be evaluated whether you perform the procedure on a person or a manikin.

It is very important that you remember to perform the beginning and ending procedure steps when appropriate. These steps include showing that you respect the patient by explaining the procedure and providing privacy. It is also imperative that you identify the patient every time by checking the identification bracelet.

Some other guidelines for taking the skills test are:

- Wear a wristwatch with a secondhand so you're prepared to take the patient's vital signs.
- Use good body mechanics when performing all procedures.
- Remember to observe standard precautions.
- Make sure the call button is within the patient's reach when you finish each procedure.
- Make sure the side rails are up when you finish each procedure or leave the patient's side.

As you prepare for your tests and for your career as a nursing assistant, remember that your job is a very important one and one that you can be proud of. You will not only be helping people but you will also be making your community a better place in which to live.

After you successfully demonstrate each procedure on the following list, have your instructor initial and date the appropriate skill.

CHAPTER 5 SKILLS

Procedure 5–1
Handwashing

Initials	Date

Procedure 5–2
Removing Gloves

Initials	Date

Procedure 5–3
Wearing a Face Mask

Initials	Date

Procedure 5–4
Applying a Gown

Initials	Date

Procedure 5–5
Removing a Gown

Initials	Date

Procedure 5–6
Terminal Cleaning of the
Patient Unit

Initials	Date

CHAPTER 6 SKILLS

Procedure 6–1
Applying a Vest Restraint

Initials	Date

Procedure 6–2
Applying a Waist Restraint

Initials	Date

CHAPTER 7 SKILL

Procedure 7–1
The Heimlich Maneuver
and Finger Sweep

Initials	Date

CHAPTER 9 SKILLS

Procedure 9–1
Measuring Oral Temperature

Initials	Date

Procedure 9–2
Measuring Rectal
Temperature

Initials	Date

Procedure 9–3
Measuring Axillary or Groin
Temperature

Initials	Date

Procedure 9–4
Measuring Temperature with an
Electronic Thermometer

Initials	Date

Procedure 9–5
Measuring the Radial Pulse Rate

Initials	Date

Procedure 9–6
Measuring the Apical Pulse Rate

Initials	Date

Procedure 9–7
Measuring the Respiratory Rate

Initials	Date

Procedure 9–8
Measuring Blood Pressure

Initials	Date

Procedure 9–9
Measuring Weight and Height

Initials	Date

CHAPTER 10 SKILLS

Procedure 10–1
Moving a Patient Up in Bed

Initials	Date

Procedure 10–2
Moving a Helpless Patient Up in Bed
(Using a Turning Sheet)

Initials	Date

Procedure 10–3
Turning a Patient Toward You

Initials	Date

Procedure 10–4
Turning a Patient Away from You

Initials	Date

Procedure 10–5
Logrolling a Patient

Initials	Date

Procedure 10–6
Assisting a Patient to the Edge
of the Bed (Dangling)

_____ _____
Initials   Date

Procedure 10–7
Transferring a Patient
from a Bed to a Chair

_____ _____
Initials   Date

Procedure 10–8
Using a Mechanical Lift

_____ _____
Initials   Date

Procedure 10–9
Assisting to Ambulate
Using a Cane or Walker

_____ _____
Initials   Date

Procedure 10–10
Assisting to Ambulate with a
Gait Belt

_____ _____
Initials   Date

Procedure 10–11
Care of a Falling Patient

_____ _____
Initials   Date

CHAPTER 12 SKILLS

Procedure 12–1
Making a Closed Bed

_____ _____
Initials   Date

Procedure 12–2
Opening a Closed Bed

_____ _____
Initials   Date

Procedure 12–3
Making an Occupied Bed

_____ _____
Initials   Date

Procedure 12–4
Making a Surgical Bed

_____ _____
Initials   Date

CHAPTER 13 SKILLS

Procedure 13–1
Giving a Complete Bed Bath

_____ _____
Initials   Date

Procedure 13–2
Giving a Partial Bed Bath

_____ _____
Initials   Date

Procedure 13–3
Assisting with a Tub Bath
or Shower

_____ _____
Initials   Date

Procedure 13–4
Giving a Bed Shampoo

Initials	Date

Procedure 13–5
Assisting with Routine
Oral Hygiene

Initials	Date

Procedure 13–6
Providing Oral Hygiene
for an Unconscious Patient

Initials	Date

Procedure 13–7
Assisting with Denture Care

Initials	Date

Procedure 13–8
Shaving a Male Patient

Initials	Date

Procedure 13–9
Assisting with Daily Hair Care

Initials	Date

Procedure 13–10
Giving Nail Care

Initials	Date

Procedure 13–11
Giving a Back Rub

Initials	Date

CHAPTER 15 SKILLS

Procedure 15–1
Serving Food

Initials	Date

Procedure 15–2
Feeding a Dependent Patient

Initials	Date

Procedure 15–3
Measuring and Recording
Fluid Intake

Initials	Date

Procedure 15–4
Measuring and Recording
Fluid Output

Initials	Date

CHAPTER 16 SKILLS

Procedure 16–1
Assisting with Use of a Urinal

Initials	Date

Procedure 16–2
Assisting with Use of a Bedpan

Initials	Date

Procedure 16–3
Assisting with Use of a
Bedside Commode

Initials	Date

Procedure 16–4
Assisting the Patient to the
Bathroom

Initials	Date

Procedure 16–5
Giving Perineal Care

Initials	Date

Procedure 16–6
Providing Catheter Care

Initials	Date

Procedure 16–7
Emptying the Urine Drainage Bag

Initials	Date

CHAPTER 17 SKILLS

Procedure 17–1
Collecting a Routine Urine
Specimen

Initials	Date

Procedure 17–2
Collecting a Stool Specimen

Initials	Date

Procedure 17–3
Collecting a Sputum Specimen

Initials	Date

CHAPTER 18 SKILLS

Procedure 18–1
Providing AM Care

Initials	Date

Procedure 18–2
Providing PM Care

Initials	Date

CHAPTER 19 SKILL

Procedure 19–1
Performing
Range-of-Motion Exercises

Initials	Date

CHAPTER 20 SKILLS

Procedure 20–1
Applying a Dry Cold Treatment

Initials	Date

Procedure 20–2
Applying an Aquamatic Pad

Initials	Date

Procedure 20–3
Assisting with a Sitz Bath

Initials	Date

Procedure 20–4
Giving a Commercial Cleansing
Enema

Initials	Date

Procedure 20–5
Giving a Commercial
Oil-Retention Enema

Initials	Date

Procedure 20–6
Giving a Cleansing Enema

Initials	Date

Procedure 20–7
Using the Disposable Rectal Tube
with Connected Flatus Bag

Initials	Date

CHAPTER 21 SKILLS

Procedure 21–1
Shaving a Patient Before Surgery

Initials	Date

Procedure 21–2
Assisting with Deep-Breathing
Exercises

Initials	Date

Procedure 21–3
Applying Elasticized Stockings

Initials	Date

Procedure 21–4
Assisting the Patient
with Initial Ambulation

Initials	Date

CHAPTER 24 SKILL

Procedure 24–1
Providing Postmortem Care

Initials	Date

Chapter 1 • Learning Activities

MediaLink

Additional free, interactive resources for this chapter can be found on the Student CD-ROM accompanying this book and on the Companion Website at **www.prenhall.com/pulliam**. Click on Chapter 1 to select activities for this chapter.

CD-ROM
Audio Glossary
Certification Exam Review
Animations/Videos:
   Reporting Upwards

Companion Website
Audio Glossary   Matching
Certification Exam Review   Study Tips
Case Studies   MediaLink
Challenge Your Knowledge

Introduction to Health Care

1. Two common purposes that health care facilities share are listed below. What are three additional common purposes?

   1. To prevent disease.

   2. To promote medical research.

   3. _____

   4. _____

   5. _____

2. What are the six main types of health care organizations that employ nursing assistants?

   1. _____

   2. _____

   3. _____

   4. _____

   5. _____

   6. _____

3. A new orderly has just started working as part of your team. He tells you that he has heard several nurses using the terms *acute* and *chronic* when referring to illnesses. He asks you to explain what they mean. What would you say?

   _____

   _____

4. Your elderly aunt is no longer able to care for herself. What type of health care facility would be able to help meet her needs?

_____

5. In addition to the elderly, what two groups of people receive care at long-term care facilities?

   1. _____

   2. _____

6. Name two ways hospice care can be provided to the dying patient and his or her family.

   1. _____

   2. _____

7. A patient tells you that her physician has recommended that she leave the hospital and receive care from a home health agency. She asks you to explain what that is. What can you tell her?

_____

_____

_____

8. Your team leader tells you that you need to get an organizational chart to study the facility's chain of command. What is a chain of command? Why is it helpful in understanding how your facility is organized?

_____

_____

9. In your health care facility, you should know where to find patient units and the staff bulletin board. What are three other things you should be able to locate?

   1. _____

   2. _____

   3. _____

10. In your health care facility, you work with a group of professionals and nonprofessionals to help plan for and meet patients' needs. What is this group called?

_____

11. If you wanted to become a Licensed Practical Nurse (LPN), or Licensed Vocational Nurse (LVN), what training would you need?

_____

_____

12. The three descriptions below explain how nursing care is organized in three different health care facilities. After each description, tell whether the organization is for primary nursing, team nursing, or functional nursing.

   1. In this facility, a head nurse directs the nursing staff in caring for patients. This nurse also assigns specific duties to nursing staff members.

   _____

   2. In this facility, a registered nurse plans and implements the care of seven patients. When this nurse isn't on duty, other nursing staff members help care for the patients.

   _____

   3. In this facility, the nursing staff is divided into teams. Each team has a leader who assigns duties to each member.

   _____

13. Listed below is one thing the patient care plan includes. What are two other things included in the care plan?

   1. The nursing diagnosis.

   2. _____

   3. _____

14. You have just gotten a job at a city hospital. A friend of yours works as a nursing assistant in another hospital in the city. He tells you that you should come to him if you have any questions about policies or procedures. Why isn't that a good idea?

   _____

   _____

15. Listed below are two of the tasks you will perform in your job as a nursing assistant. What are two more tasks?

   1. Take direction from RNs and LPNs to carry out the care plan for the patient.

   2. Provide physical and emotional support to patients.

   3. _____

   4. _____

   _____
   Signature   **Date**

MediaLink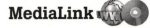

Additional free, interactive resources for this chapter can be found on the Student CD-ROM accompanying this book and on the Companion Website at **www.prenhall.com/pulliam**. Click on Chapter 2 to select activities for this chapter.

CD-ROM	**Companion Website**	
Audio Glossary	Audio Glossary	Matching
Certification Exam Review	Certification Exam Review	Study Tips
Animations/Videos:	Case Studies	MediaLink
Job of the Nursing	Challenge Your Knowledge	
Assistant		

The Nursing Assistant

1. Listed below are three duties you will have as a nursing assistant. What are three other duties?

    1. Helping patients with personal needs.

    2. Helping to make patients physically comfortable and assisting them with mobility and activity needs.

    3. Attending to patients' psychological comfort and social and cultural needs.

    4. _____

    5. _____

    6. _____

2. You are good friends with a patient's sister. Your friend is very worried about her brother and asks you what type of treatment he's receiving. What would you tell her? Why?

    _____

    _____

3. Listed below are four tasks that aren't within your scope of practice. What are four other tasks you aren't legally permitted to perform?

1. Telling anyone about a patient's diagnosis or treatment.

2. Doing something you're not properly trained to do.

3. Performing sterile procedures.

4. Inserting or removing tubes from a patient's body.

5. _____

6. _____

7. _____

8. _____

4. Your next-door neighbor tells you that her daughter wants to become a nursing assistant. She asks you what you have to do to become certified. What would you tell her?

_____

_____

5. A co-worker took 2½ years off after she had a baby. Can she come back to work right away? Why or why not?

_____

_____

6. What policy deals with patient rights?

_____

7. A patient of yours has refused to have surgery, and he is preparing to leave the hospital. Does anyone have the legal right to keep him there?

_____

8. Standards of care are based on laws. What other three things are they based on?

1. _____

2. _____

3. _____

9. Negligence is an unintentional wrong that causes harm to a patient. Listed below are two ways you can harm a patient and be considered negligent. What are two others?

1. Disregard a supervisor's instructions.

2. Perform a task incorrectly or unsafely.

3. _____

4. _____

10. The three following situations involve behavior that may or may not be considered negligent. After each description, tell whether the nursing assistant was negligent. Then explain your answer.

1. While the nursing assistant was helping a patient to his bed, the patient slipped on a wet spot on the floor and hurt his ankle. The nursing assistant had been very careful, but hadn't seen the wet spot.

_____

_____

2. The head nurse tells the nursing assistant to collect a patient's urine specimen. The nursing assistant has never done that before, but she's afraid to tell that to the nurse. When she collects the specimen, she contaminates it by touching the inside of the specimen container.

_____

_____

3. The nursing assistant attempts to transfer a patient into a wheelchair. Before moving the patient, the nursing assistant discovers that the brakes on the wheelchair are broken. He decides that he can hold the wheelchair steady on his own. During the transfer, the wheelchair rolls and the patient falls.

_____

_____

11. If a nursing assistant intentionally causes harm to a patient, a form of abuse has been committed. After each statement that follows, write which type of abuse the nursing assistant is guilty of.

1. The nursing assistant makes fun of a patient's weight.

_____

2. The nursing assistant decides to apply a restraint to a patient who has been trying to climb out of bed all shift. There isn't a doctor's order for the restraint.

_____

3. The nursing assistant screams at the patient for soiling her bed.

_____

12. Nursing assistants have a responsibility to keep the information in patients' charts confidential. What other responsibility do they have concerning charts?

_____

13. Listed below is one reason why it is important that nursing assistants maintain their personal health, hygiene, and appearance. What are two other reasons?

1. Their health and hygiene practices set an example for others.

2. _____

3. _____

14. Nursing assistants may be exposed to many different disease-causing organisms during the performance of job duties. Your employer will instruct you on the appropriate personal protective equipment to use and precautions to take to reduce your risk of exposure. List two viruses that are of special concern to health care workers, including nursing assistants.

1. _____

2. _____

_____

Signature   **Date**

MediaLink

Additional free, interactive resources for this chapter can be found on the Student CD-ROM accompanying this book and on the Companion Website at **www.prenhall.com/pulliam**. Click on Chapter 3 to select activities for this chapter.

CD-ROM	Companion Website	
Audio Glossary	Audio Glossary	Matching
Certification Exam Review	Certification Exam Review	Study Tips
Animations/Videos:	Case Studies	MediaLink
Good and Bad	Challenge Your Knowledge	
Communication Skills		

Communication and Interpersonal Skills

1. Patience and empathy are two important interpersonal skills. What are four more?

    1. _____

    2. _____

    3. _____

    4. _____

2. Listed below is one element of the communications process. What are the three other basic elements?

    1. The sender.

    2. _____

    3. _____

    4. _____

3. Read the situations below. Then write which element of the communication process was ineffective.

   1. Your supervisor tells you to give the patient in Room 68 a bed bath. You listen and go to do the task. When you get to the room, you realize you forgot to ask which patient she meant.

   _____

   2. You tell a patient he can't smoke in his room. He doesn't stop because he can't understand you—he doesn't speak English.

   _____

   3. You go to the nurse's station to report your patient's complaint of pain. The nurse is on the phone, but she looks up so you think she's acknowledging you. You pass on the message, and she nods her head. You leave the desk to attend to another patient. At the end of your shift, the nurse stops you and asks you what you wanted earlier.

   _____

4. Read each situation below. Write whether the situation illustrates verbal or nonverbal communication.

   1. The patient is smiling and sitting up straight.

   _____

   2. The nurse has her hands on her hips and an angry expression on her face.

   _____

   3. The physician listens to the patient complain about his back.

   _____

5. Whenever you try to tell your team leader about an observation, he interrupts you. What skill does he lack?

   _____

6. To receive messages properly, you need to have good listening skills. List three things a skilled listener would do.

   1. _____

   2. _____

   3. _____

7. To communicate well with others, you need to speak clearly. What are three other guidelines for effective communication?

   1. _____

   2. _____

   3. _____

8. You are walking down the hall when you see the call-light signal blink on for a patient's room. What should you do?

_____

_____

_____

_____

9. Listed below are two guidelines to follow when you communicate with people over the telephone. What are three others?

1. Identify yourself.

2. Speak clearly.

3. _____

4. _____

5. _____

10. Read the description below. After each description, write whether it is an example of objective data or subjective data.

1. A patient tells you that he feels sick to his stomach.

_____

2. You feel a lump under a patient's skin.

_____

3. You report that a patient didn't eat well today.

_____

4. A patient complains of dizziness.

_____

11. Which of your senses will you use to observe patients and collect objective data?

1. _____

2. _____

3. _____

4. _____

12. There are many patient conditions that you need to report to your supervisor immediately. List four of the nine possible conditions.

1. _____

2. _____

3. _____

4. _____

13. When you record information in a patient's chart, what are the most important principles?

_____

14. Describe the differences between word roots, prefixes, and suffixes.

_____

_____

_____

_____

Signature   **Date**

MediaLink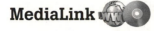

Additional free, interactive resources for this chapter can be found on the Student CD-ROM accompanying this book and on the Companion Website at **www.prenhall.com/pulliam**. Click on Chapter 4 to select activities for this chapter.

CD-ROM	**Companion Website**	
Audio Glossary	Audio Glossary	Matching
Certification Exam Review	Certification Exam Review	Study Tips
Animations/Videos:	Case Studies	MediaLink
Interacting with the Patient's Family	Challenge Your Knowledge	

Relating to Your Patients

1. Listed below is one thing you need to know to understand your patients' situation and needs. What are two others?

    1. Patients are people, not a set of symptoms.

    2. _____

    3. _____

2. Fill in the two basic needs missing from Maslow's hierarchy below.

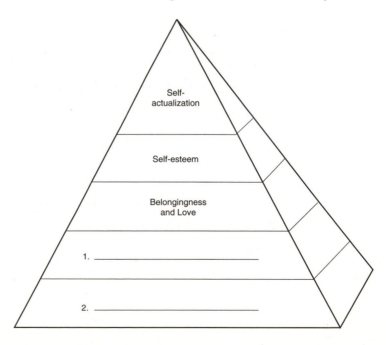

3. A middle-aged patient tells you that he's worried about his upcoming operation. What should you do?

_____

_____

4. Patients in long-term care facilities may experience feelings of loss. What are three other feelings they may experience?

1. _____

2. _____

3. _____

5. An elderly patient is very upset because her only son is moving away. She wants to be near him but she doesn't want to leave the nursing home because she has made a lot of friends there. What should you do to help her with her problem?

_____

_____

6. Listed below are two factors that could affect your patients' behavior. What are three other factors?

1. Unmet needs.

2. Life experiences, attitudes, and prejudices.

3. _____

4. _____

5. _____

7. In your health care facility, patients share rooms. A patient has come to you and complained that he's unhappy with his new roommate because he speaks another language. He says that people in this country ought to speak English if they want to live here. What has probably caused his negative attitude?

_____

8. In the preceding situation, what might you say the English-speaking patient is guilty of?

_____

9. Choose one age group, and list the communication, comfort, and safety care considerations that apply.

1. Group: _____

2. Communication: _____

_____

_____

3. Comfort:_____

_____

_____

4. Safety: _____

_____

_____

10. Self-centered behavior and crying are two types of difficult behavior you may have to cope with. What are three other types?

    1. _____

    2. _____

    3. _____

11. A new patient is constantly pushing the call button so you'll come to her. Most of the time, she doesn't need anything except your attention. What should you do?

_____

_____

12. A patient does not want you to give him a bed bath. In fact, he gets so mad as you prepare the bath that he hits you and throws water on you. What should you do?

_____

_____

13. Many times, health care workers feel angry and frustrated with patients. Listed below is an example of an inappropriate response to a patient. List three other examples of behavior that is unacceptable when caring for patients.

    1. Shouting at the patient.

    2. _____

    3. _____

    4. _____

14. A patient's wife has asked you why her husband is hooked up to an intravenous tube. You know the answer. Do you tell her? Explain your answer.

_____

_____

15. If patients have different religious beliefs than you do, how should you react to them?

_____

_____

16. A patient who cannot speak English has just been admitted to a unit you are responsible for. What should you do?

_____

_____

17. Fill in the blanks in the paragraph below to explain how you should communicate with a patient who has diminished sight.

Identify (1) _____ when you enter the patient's room. Explain all (2) _____. Have the patient wear (3) _____, and clean them if necessary. Allow the patient to touch (4) _____ or (5) _____ if necessary.

_____

Signature   **Date**

Chapter 5 • Learning Activities

MediaLink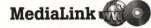

Additional free, interactive resources for this chapter can be found on the Student CD-ROM accompanying this book and on the Companion Website at **www.prenhall.com/ pulliam**. Click on Chapter 5 to select activities for this chapter.

CD-ROM
Audio Glossary
Certification Exam Review
Animations/Videos:
  Applying a Mask;
  Gowning; Removing
  Gloves; Hand
  Hygiene

Companion Website
Audio Glossary   Matching
Certification Exam Review   Study Tips
Case Studies   MediaLink
Challenge Your Knowledge

Infection Control

1. What is the most basic and important procedure in nursing care?

   _____

2. Can you get rid of all microorganisms if you keep things clean? Explain your answer.

   _____

   _____

3. Listed below is one type of microorganism that causes diseases. What are three other common types?

   1. Bacteria

   2. _____

   3. _____

   4. _____

4. Pathogens survive best under certain conditions. Fill in the blanks below to describe those conditions.

   Bacteria grow best in the remains of (1) _____ and in

   (2) _____ places. High temperature (3) _____ most

   bacteria. Some bacteria require (4) _____ and some do not.

   (5) _____ helps the development of bacteria. Bacteria may live on

   dead or living matter or (6) _____.

5. Read the situations below. Then tell which of the five basic modes of transmission for infectious diseases is being described.

1. One person sneezes and another inhales the infectious particles.

_____

2. Two people kiss and transmit the infection.

_____

3. A tick carries the disease.

_____

6. The diagram below describes the chain of infection. Fill in each blank with the appropriate term from the following list: causative agent, mode of transmission, portal of entry, portal of exit, reservoir of the agent, susceptible host.

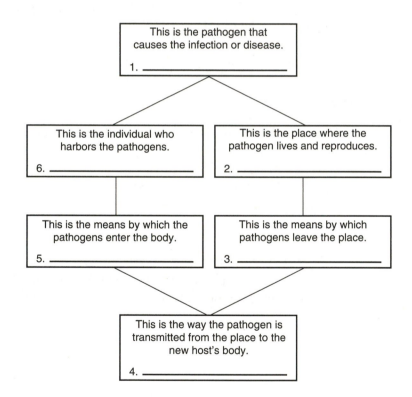

This is the pathogen that causes the infection or disease.

1. _____

This is the individual who harbors the pathogens.

6. _____

This is the place where the pathogen lives and reproduces.

2. _____

This is the means by which the pathogens enter the body.

5. _____

This is the means by which pathogens leave the place.

3. _____

This is the way the pathogen is transmitted from the place to the new host's body.

4. _____

7. List four of the body's defenses that defend it from infection.

1. _____

2. _____

3. _____

4. _____

8. A patient's abdominal incision appears more red and swollen today. He also has a fever. What might this signal? What should you do?

_____

_____

9. Write whether the following objects are sterile, clean, or dirty.

1. An object not contaminated by pathogens.

_____

2. A contaminated object.

_____

3. An object free from all microorganisms.

_____

10. What should you do if you cut yourself while you're at work?

_____

11. If clean linen falls to the floor in a patient's room, can you still use it to make that patient's bed? Why or why not?

_____

12. Barriers, or personal protective equipment, include what items?

1. _____

2. _____

3. _____

4. _____

13. You will be performing a procedure during which you may come in contact with the patient's body fluids. In fact, the fluids may even spatter or splash you. What standard precautions should you take?

_____

_____

14. List three of the many times you will need to wash your hands.

1. _____

2. _____

3. _____

15. Listed below are two of the times you will need to wear gloves. What are three others?

1. When you may have contact with a patient's blood or body fluids.

2. When you collect or transport a specimen.

3. _____

4. _____

5. _____

16. What are two reasons why patients are placed on transmission-based precautions?

_____

_____

_____

Signature   **Date**

MediaLink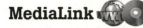

Additional free, interactive resources for this chapter can be found on the Student CD-ROM accompanying this book and on the Companion Website at **www.prenhall.com/pulliam**. Click on Chapter 6 to select activities for this chapter.

CD-ROM
Audio Glossary
Certification Exam Review
Animations/Videos:
  General Safety Rules;
  Applying a Vest
  Restraint; Applying a
  Waist Restraint

Companion Website
Audio Glossary
Certification Exam Review
Case Studies
Challenge Your Knowledge

Matching
Study Tips
MediaLink

Environmental Safety, Accident Prevention, and Disaster Plans

1. Why are some potential hazards unique to hospitals and long-term care facilities?

   _____

   _____

2. What is the patient's primary way to signal a problem?

   _____

3. Listed below are three safety rules that apply in any health care setting. What are four other safety rules?

   1. Identify the patient.

   2. Take care in halls and on stairs.

   3. Use equipment safely.

   4. _____

   5. _____

   6. _____

   7. _____

4. You have been assigned to a new wing of the health care facility. The head nurse tells you that many of the patients are at risk of falling. What are some things you can do to prevent patients from falling?

   _____

   _____

   _____

5. Listed below are two ways to prevent burns in health care settings. What are three other ways to prevent them?

1. Make sure patients follow the smoking policy.

2. Test bath or shower water carefully.

3. _____

4. _____

5. _____

6. If you cannot read the label on a medicine dropper, what should you do?

_____

7. Listed below is one way that you can help prevent suffocation. What are three other ways?

1. Never leave a patient unattended in a bathtub.

2. _____

3. _____

4. _____

8. What are the three basic steps to follow when you lift a heavy object from the floor?

1. _____

2. _____

3. _____

9. You need to move a bedside chair into a patient's unit. Explain why you should use proper body mechanics. Then describe how you would use proper body mechanics while lifting and moving the chair.

_____

_____

_____

_____

10. List three of the most common types of restraints.

1. _____

2. _____

3. _____

11. One of your patients keeps slipping down in her bedside chair while you tend to other patients. You're afraid that she will fall out and injure herself. Another nursing assistant suggests that you put a waist restraint on the patient to keep her safe. What should you do? Why?

_____

_____

_____

_____

12. How frequently do you have to check on patients with restraints? What should you check?

_____

_____

13. How frequently and for how long do you have to remove restraints? What should you do for the patient when the restraint is removed?

_____

_____

14. List the three things needed to start a fire.

1. _____

2. _____

3. _____

15. Listed below is one measure you can take to be prepared in case a fire breaks out. What are three others?

1. Know your facility's floor plan and each person's responsibility.

2. _____

3. _____

4. _____

16. When you enter a patient's room, you see that the air-conditioning unit is smoking. What should you do?

_____

_____

_____
Signature   **Date**

MediaLink

Additional free, interactive resources for this chapter can be found on the Student CD-ROM accompanying this book and on the Companion Website at **www.prenhall.com/ pulliam**. Click on Chapter 7 to select activities for this chapter.

CD-ROM	**Companion Website**	
Audio Glossary	Audio Glossary	Matching
Certification Exam Review	Certification Exam Review	Study Tips
Animations/Videos:	Case Studies	MediaLink
Heimlich Maneuver	Challenge Your Knowledge	

Emergency Situations

1. Listed below are three life-threatening situations. What are three more?

   1. Choking.

   2. No breathing.

   3. No pulse.

   4. _____

   5. _____

   6. _____

2. Upon entering a patient's room, you discover that he is bleeding badly. How should you respond to this emergency situation?

   _____

   _____

3. In the preceding situation, you have to dial 911 to summon emergency help. What information will you need to give the dispatcher?

   _____

   _____

4. Before emergency help arrives, you must prioritize tasks. How can you do that?

   _____

   _____

5. You see that *no code* is written on your patient's chart. What does it mean?

   _____

   _____

6. List four of the seven signs that indicate that a patient's heartbeat and breathing have stopped.

   1. _____

   2. _____

   3. _____

   4. _____

7. What is CPR and what does it combine?

   _____

   _____

8. What are the ABCs of CPR?

   A _____

   B _____

   C _____

9. How can you learn CPR?

   _____

   _____

10. Listed below are two important points to remember when using an automatic external defibrillator (AED). What are two more?

    1. There should be no physical contact with the patient during the analysis and shock.

    2. The "apex" pad will be applied to the left side of the chest, with the top margin several inches below the left armpit.

    3. _____

    4. _____

11. You find a patient in what appears to be an unconscious state. What should you do?

    _____

    _____

    _____

12. What is the most common cause of choking in adults?

    _____

13. Read each description and tell whether the patient has a partial blockage or a complete blockage.

    1. The patient is clutching his throat and cannot speak.

    _____

2. The patient is coughing and wheezing as he breathes.

_____

14. Listed below are three possible causes of seizures. What are two more?

1. Head injury.

2. Stroke.

3. Infection or high fever.

4. _____

5. _____

15. Read each description below and tell whether the patient is having a grand mal seizure or petit mal seizure.

1. The patient has lost consciousness and his body is rigid.

_____

2. The patient is staring into space and her facial muscles are twitching.

_____

16. Listed below are the first four actions you would take if you observed a patient having a seizure. What are the next four?

1. Call for help.

2. Stay with the patient.

3. Protect the patient from injury.

4. Don't restrain the patient or place anything in the patient's mouth.

5. _____

6. _____

7. _____

8. _____

17. While a patient was getting out of bed, she caught her foot in the sheet and fell. What should you do?

_____

_____

_____
Signature   **Date**

MediaLink

Additional free, interactive resources for this chapter can be found on the Student CD-ROM accompanying this book and on the Companion Website at **www.prenhall.com/ pulliam**. Click on Chapter 8 to select activities for this chapter.

CD-ROM
Audio Glossary
Certification Exam Review
Animations/Videos:
  Respiratory System;
  Circulatory System;
  Heart; Major Veins
  and Arteries; Perform
  a Blood Glucose
  Evaluation

Companion Website
Audio Glossary
Certification Exam Review
Case Studies
Challenge Your Knowledge

Matching
Study Tips
MediaLink

Body Systems and Common Diseases

1. Why do you need to know basic anatomy and physiology?

   _____

   _____

2. On the numbered answer lines below, fill in the three descriptions of the anatomical terms used to describe where body parts are located.

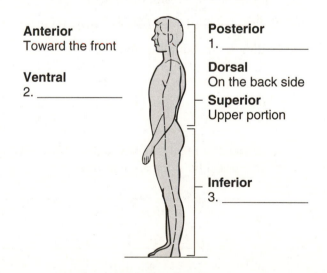

Anterior
Toward the front

Ventral
2. _____

Posterior
1. _____

Dorsal
On the back side

Superior
Upper portion

Inferior
3. _____

3. The paragraph below describes the four basic levels that make up the body's structure. Fill in each blank with the appropriate term from the chapter.

The basic units in all living things are (1) _____. Groups of

these basic units combine to form (2) _____. Tissues are

grouped together to form (3) _____. A (4) _____ is a

group of organs that works together to carry out a primary body function.

4. There are four basic kinds of tissue: epithelial, connective, muscle, and nerve. Each has a different function. Read the description of a tissue's function below and tell which kind of tissue it is.

1. Holds other tissues together.

_____

2. Receives sensations.

_____

3. Regulates body functions.

_____

4. Enables the body to move.

_____

5. What is the body process that keeps blood pressure, body temperature, and fluid balance constant or within certain limits?

_____

6. What is the difference between growth and development?

_____

_____

7. Listed below are two factors that influence how a person grows and develops. What are three other factors?

1. Characteristics inherited from parents.

2. The surrounding environment.

3. _____

4. _____

5. _____

8. If you observe a patient coughing or vomiting, you should notify your supervisor immediately. What are four other possible signs or symptoms of disease?

1. _____

2. _____

3. _____

4. _____

9. How is the HIV/AIDS virus transmitted?

_____

_____

10. Read each description below of a person infected with the AIDS virus. Write which stage of the disease the person is in: HIV-positive, pre-AIDS, or AIDS.

    1. This person has night sweats and diarrhea.

    _____

    2. This person has Kaposi's sarcoma.

    _____

    3. This person's health seems to be unaffected.

    _____

11. Why are standard precautions used when caring for all patients, not just HIV-positive or AIDS patients?

_____

_____

12. Listed below are three of the warning signs of cancer that begin to spell *CAUTION*. What are the other four signs?

    C—Change in bowel or bladder habits.

    A—A sore that doesn't heal.

    U—Unusual bleeding or discharge.

    T— _____

    I— _____

    O— _____

    N— _____

13. Listed below is one function of each of the following nine systems of the body: respiratory, circulatory, gastrointestinal, urinary, endocrine, reproductive, integumentary, musculoskeletal, and nervous. After each function, tell which system it describes. The first one has been done for you.

    1. This system takes blood to the cells and carries waste products away from the cells.

       The circulatory system.

    2. This system excretes liquid waste products that are removed from the blood.

    _____

3. This system brings oxygen into the body and eliminates carbon dioxide.

_____

4. This system provides a framework for the body and allows it to move.

_____

5. This system breaks down food and removes solid waste products that result from the digestive process.

_____

6. This system produces reproductive cells.

_____

7. This system secretes hormones that regulate body functions.

_____

8. This system controls and coordinates all functions of the body.

_____

9. This system protects the inside of the body against injury and disease.

_____

14. You have been asked to care for a patient with breathing problems. How should you care for this patient?

_____

_____

_____

15. What types of disease are the leading causes of death in the United States?

_____

16. What is your primary task when giving care to a heart patient?

_____

_____

17. A patient who has diabetes mellitus refuses to follow her diet. What should you do?

_____

_____

18. A patient has just had a cast put on his leg. What precautions do you need to follow when caring for his cast?

_____

_____

_____

19. A patient who has just been admitted is mentally retarded. Should you treat her any differently than other patients? Explain your answer.

_____

_____

_____

_____

Signature   **Date**

MediaLink

Additional free, interactive resources for this chapter can be found on the Student CD-ROM accompanying this book and on the Companion Website at **www.prenhall.com/ pulliam**. Click on Chapter 9 to select activities for this chapter.

CD-ROM	Companion Website	
Audio Glossary	Audio Glossary	Matching
Certification Exam Review	Certification Exam Review	Study Tips
Animations/Videos:	Case Studies	MediaLink
Measuring Blood Pressure	Challenge Your Knowledge	

Vital Signs

1. Listed below is one of the vital signs. What are three others?

   1. Body temperature.

   2. _____

   3. _____

   4. _____

2. What are baseline measurements?

   _____

   _____

3. How do you know how often to take a patient's vital signs?

   _____

4. You get an abnormally low blood pressure reading on one of your patients. What should you do?

   _____

5. List four of the factors that affect a person's body temperature.

   1. _____

   2. _____

   3. _____

   4. _____

6. What are the four major methods used in health care facilities to measure body temperature?

1. _____

2. _____

3. _____

4. _____

7. Which method of measuring body temperature is the least accurate?

_____

8. What precautions should you follow before using a glass thermometer?

_____

_____

9. Listed below is one reason for not using the rectal method to take a patient's temperature. What are three others?

1. Diarrhea.

2. _____

3. _____

4. _____

10. You are taking a patient's pulse. What things do you need to observe?

_____

11. In the following situations, would you take a radial pulse or an apical pulse?

1. The patient is taking medication that affects his heart.

_____

2. The patient has a broken leg.

_____

12. You and a co-worker take a patient's apical–radial pulse. The apical pulse rate is 79. The radial pulse rate is 75. What is the pulse deficit? What should you do about it?

_____

13. You need to measure a patient's respiratory rate. How would you do it? If it were 24, would it be considered normal?

_____

_____

14. List four of the factors that can affect a person's blood pressure.

1. _____

2. _____

3. _____

4. _____

15. Your patient has just returned to her unit after taking a walk. Your supervisor has instructed you to take the patient's blood pressure. Should you take it now? Explain your answer.

_____

_____

16. When you take the patient's blood pressure, it is 140/100. Is that normal? What should you do?

_____

17. Listed below is one reason why a patient's weight is rechecked periodically in a health care facility. What are three others?

1. Medications may need to be changed if weight changes.

2. _____

3. _____

4. _____

18. The chart below shows normal ranges for temperature, pulse rates, and blood pressure. Fill in the blanks in the chart to complete the information.

Normal Ranges

Temperature Method	Body Temperature
Oral	97.6°F–99.6°F
1. _____	98.6°F–100.6°F
Axillary	96.6°F–98.6°F
Age Group	**Pulse Rates per Minute**
2. _____	80–120
Adult Years	60–100
Later Years	3. _____
Age Group	**Systolic Blood Pressure**
Adult	90–140 mm Hg
4. _____	140–160 mm Hg
Age Group	**Diastolic Blood Pressure**
Adult	60–90 mm Hg
Older Adult	5. _____

_____

Signature   **Date**

Chapter 10 • Learning Activities

Positioning, Moving, and Ambulation

1. Listed below are two important points to remember when positioning, moving, or transporting a patient. What are four other points to remember?

   1. Use correct body alignment.

   2. Reduce friction and shearing between the patient's skin and sheets whenever possible.

   3. _____

   4. _____

   5. _____

   6. _____

2. The paragraph below discusses devices that make patients more secure and comfortable when they are in bed and during moves. Fill in each blank with the appropriate term.

   (1) _____ in a variety of sizes are used to support the body in

   a certain position or to prevent a patient from rolling over. Other

   support devices are folded or rolled towels or blankets. One particular type of support, called a (2) _____, is made from a blanket

rolled and tucked along patients' sides to prevent hip rotation. A

(3) _____ is used to add extra support to a mattress or to

prevent it from sagging. Footdrop can be prevented by using a

(4) _____. To move a helpless patient in bed, (5) _____

should be used.

3. You need to sponge-bathe a patient who has a spinal cord injury caused in a car accident. What procedure should you use to turn her in bed? Briefly describe this procedure.

    _____

    _____

    _____

    _____

4. A patient does not want to get out of bed and walk around. What four benefits can you tell him are gained from getting out of bed and sitting in a chair or walking?

    1. _____

    2. _____

    3. _____

    4. _____

5. A patient with hepatitis has not been out of bed for nearly 2 weeks. She is now ready to get out of bed. What steps should you take to assist her in getting up and, perhaps, walking?

    _____

    _____

    _____

    _____

6. Your supervisor has instructed you to use a transfer belt to move a patient from her bed to a chair. What do you need to do when using the belt?

    _____

    _____

    _____

7. What is a stretcher? What are two other names for this device?

    _____

    _____

44

8. A helpless patient who weighs 230 pounds needs help to get out of bed and into a wheelchair. How would you handle this situation?

_____

_____

_____

9. When you transport a patient by wheelchair or stretcher, you need to reassure the patient. List three other guidelines you should keep in mind.

1. _____

2. _____

3. _____

10. What special considerations would you need to observe if you were transporting a person on a stretcher in an elevator?

_____

_____

11. The following mechanical aids are used for ambulation. Label each aid on the line provided.

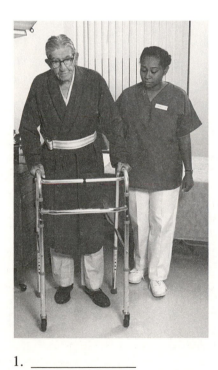

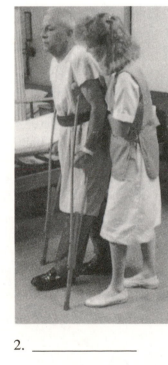

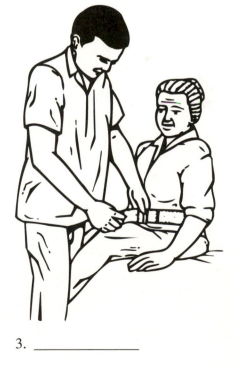

1. _____   2. _____   3. _____

12. The safety guidelines below are used when assisting a patient with ambulation. List three others.

1. Follow the rules for good body mechanics.

2. Frequently check walking aids to make sure they are in good repair.

3. _____

4. _____

5. _____

13. To help prevent patients from falling and injuring themselves, you need to be aware that some patients are more prone to falls than others. In what two situations do patients need to be watched very closely?

1. _____

2. _____

_____

Signature   **Date**

46

Chapter 11 • Learning Activities

MediaLink

Additional free, interactive resources for this chapter can be found on the Student CD-ROM accompanying this book and on the Companion Website at **www.prenhall.com/pulliam**. Click on Chapter 11 to select activities for this chapter.

CD-ROM	**Companion Website**	
Audio Glossary	Audio Glossary	Matching
Certification Exam Review	Certification Exam Review	Study Tips
Animations/Videos:	Case Studies	MediaLink
Admission; Transfer; Discharge	Challenge Your Knowledge	

Admission, Transfer, and Discharge

1. Each statement below refers to either the admission, transfer, or discharge of a patient. After each one, name the procedure.

   1. A patient is leaving the facility and going home.

      _____

   2. A patient is entering a long-term care facility.

      _____

   3. A patient is moving from intensive care to a regular unit.

      _____

2. Listed below is one situation in which the term *transfer* is used. What are two other situations in which this term is used?

   1. When a patient moves from the present patient unit to another patient unit.

   2. _____

   3. _____

3. You have just discharged a patient from your hospital who is being taken to a rehabilitation facility across the city. The patient's husband wants to know why you are using the term *discharge* and not *transfer*. What should you tell him?

   _____

   _____

4. What is the basis for Medicare or Medicaid payments to health care providers?

   _____

5. During the admission process, an elderly patient tells you that he has a living will. What should you do with this information?

   _____

6. During the admission process, nursing assistants are expected to follow the policies of the facility as well as the instructions of the nurse in charge. What are four other responsibilities that nursing assistants have during the admission process?

   1. _____

   2. _____

   3. _____

   4. _____

7. A car accident victim is being admitted to your facility. She is wearing an expensive pearl necklace. What should you do with this personal belonging?

   _____

8. Admission to a long-term care facility involves different considerations than admission to a short-term care facility. One factor that should be considered when admitting a patient to a long-term care facility is listed below. What are four other factors?

   1. The patient's feelings of loss and grief over what is being given up.

   2. _____

   3. _____

   4. _____

   5. _____

9. A patient has just asked for a different room because of noise near the nursing station. What are three other reasons a patient might be transferred?

   1. _____

   2. _____

   3. _____

10. Listed below are three of the tasks that nursing assistants perform during the transfer process. List four other tasks.

1. Follow policies and instructions of the facility.

2. Prepare the new unit.

3. Prepare the patient.

4. _____

5. _____

6. _____

7. _____

11. Who can authorize a patient's discharge?

_____

12. What is a discharge that is *against medical advice* (AMA)? Who handles such a discharge?

_____

13. Part of discharge planning may include educating the patient and family about continued care. One such educational topic concerns instructions for administration of medication. What are three other topics that would fall under the task of educating the patient and his family?

1. _____

2. _____

3. _____

14. A patient tells you she will be discharged right after lunch. How can you help this patient prepare for her discharge?

_____

_____

_____

15. What are three follow-up procedures you may have to perform after a patient has been discharged?

1. _____

2. _____

3. _____

16. A discharge procedure checklist helps nursing assistants perform their responsibilities better. Below is a partially completed checklist for discharge procedures. Fill in four tasks that a nursing assistant should perform in the event of a patient's discharge.

Discharge Procedures Checklist
(Initial each task after its completion.)
_SK_ Be sure to follow all facility policies and supervisor's instructions.
_SK_ Help the patient.
_____ 1. _____
_____ 2. _____
_____ 3. _____
_____ 4. _____

_____

Signature   **Date**

Chapter 12 • Learning Activities

MediaLink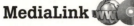

Additional free, interactive resources for this chapter can be found on the Student CD-ROM accompanying this book and on the Companion Website at **www.prenhall.com/pulliam**. Click on Chapter 12 to select activities for this chapter.

CD-ROM	Companion Website	
Audio Glossary	Audio Glossary	Matching
Certification Exam Review	Certification Exam Review	Study Tips
Animations/Videos:	Case Studies	MediaLink
Making an Occupied Bed	Challenge Your Knowledge	

The Patient's Environment

1. Listed below are two pieces of furniture typically found in the patient unit. What are three others?

   1. Bed.

   2. Overbed table.

   3. _____

   4. _____

   5. _____

2. What is the call system in a health care facility?

   _____

   _____

   _____

3. List four of the factors that affect how comfortable a patient's environment is.

   1. _____

   2. _____

   3. _____

   4. _____

4. Your supervisor has asked you to make sure that all patients have fresh drinking water and other supplies within their reach. What does he mean by "other supplies"?

_____

_____

5. What else should be within patients' reach?

_____

6. How can you provide a patient with privacy?

_____

_____

_____

7. Label the types of beds in the pictures below. One has already been done for you.

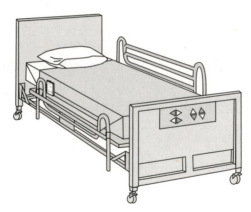 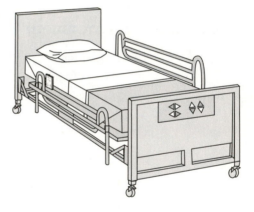

(1) Closed bed _____ (2) _____

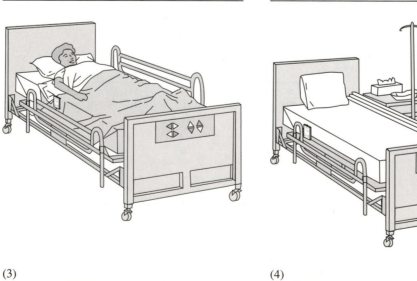

(3) _____ (4) _____

8. The patient in Room 212 has just been discharged. No new patient is scheduled to occupy the unit. What type of bed should you make?

_____

9. The patient in Room 127 will be returning to her unit soon after having gallbladder surgery. Your supervisor told you to make the bed before the patient returns. What type of bed should you make? Explain your answer.

_____

_____

_____

Signature   **Date**

Chapter 13 • Learning Activities

MediaLink

Additional free, interactive resources for this chapter can be found on the Student CD-ROM accompanying this book and on the Companion Website at **www.prenhall.com/pulliam**. Click on Chapter 13 to select activities for this chapter.

CD-ROM	Companion Website	
Audio Glossary	Audio Glossary	Matching
Certification Exam Review	Certification Exam Review	Study Tips
Animations/Videos:	Case Studies	MediaLink
Assisting with Routine Oral Hygiene	Challenge Your Knowledge	

Hygiene and Grooming

1. Listed below are three types of personal hygiene and grooming activities. What are five more?

   1. Bathing.

   2. Shampooing the hair.

   3. Oral hygiene.

   4. _____

   5. _____

   6. _____

   7. _____

   8. _____

2. What factors influence patients' personal hygiene needs and practices?

   _____

3. What four things determine which type of bath a patient receives?

   1. _____

   2. _____

   3. _____

   4. _____

4. Your supervisor has asked you to give a patient a partial sponge bath. In addition to the face and hands, what other parts of the patient's body do you need to wash?

_____

5. While you are bathing a patient, you observe a rash on his upper arm. What should you do?

_____

6. As one of your first tasks at your new job at a nursing home, you have been asked to help residents dress in the morning. What should you do?

_____

_____

7. While you are in the tub room with a patient who is bathing, a co-worker comes in and asks you to help her move a patient. What should you do? Explain your answer.

_____

_____

_____

8. Listed below are three conditions of patients' mouths that you should report to your supervisor. What are four more?

1. Extremely bad breath.

2. Damaged dentures.

3. Bleeding.

4. _____

5. _____

6. _____

7. _____

9. One of your patients has dentures. How often should they be cleaned?

_____

10. What should you do after assisting with patients' hair care?

_____

_____

11. What should you do before performing nail care? Why?

_____

_____

12. Three items are used during fingernail care: an orange stick, a nail clipper, and an emery board. Below each description, tell which item you should use.

1. Use this to smooth rough edges.

_____

2. Use this to cut and trim nails.

_____

3. Use this to push back cuticles.

_____

13. How do back rubs benefit patients?

_____

14. Your supervisor has asked you to observe a patient's skin closely when you give her a back rub. What type of observations should you report to your supervisor?

_____

15. The drawings below show three steps in giving a back rub. Match each of the steps with the drawing it describes.

Step 1: Apply the lotion to the patient's back with the palms of your gloved hands. Use long, smooth strokes from the buttocks to the shoulders and down the sides of the back and buttocks.

Step 2: Repeat the procedure four times with the long, smooth upward stroke and then a circular motion on the downstroke.

Step 3: Repeat again, but on the downward stroke, rub in a small circular motion with the palms of your gloved hands.

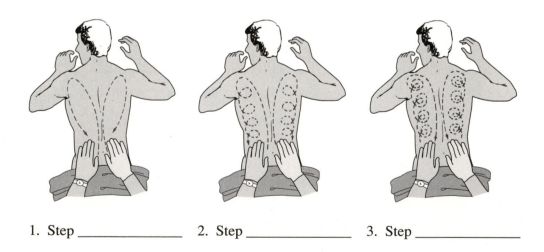

1. Step _____ 2. Step _____ 3. Step _____

16. Listed below are two tasks you need to perform when caring for hearing aids. What are three others?

1. Check the batteries regularly.

2. Check for wax buildup.

3. _____

4. _____

5. _____

_____

Signature   **Date**

MediaLink

Additional free, interactive resources for this chapter can be found on the Student CD-ROM accompanying this book and on the Companion Website at **www.prenhall.com/pulliam**. Click on Chapter 14 to select activities for this chapter.

CD-ROM	**Companion Website**	
Audio Glossary	Audio Glossary	Matching
Certification Exam Review	Certification Exam Review	Study Tips
Animations/Videos:	Case Studies	MediaLink
Preventing Skin Problems	Challenge Your Knowledge	

Special Skin Care

1. Listed below are two groups of patients who are at risk of getting decubitus ulcers. What are three other groups?

    1. The elderly.

    2. Very thin patients.

    3. _____

    4. _____

    5. _____

2. What causes decubitus ulcers?

    _____

3. Where on the body, in general, do decubitus ulcers occur most frequently?

    _____

    _____

4. List four pressure points on the body.

    1. _____

    2. _____

    3. _____

    4. _____

5. Obese patients may also develop decubitus ulcers where body parts rub together, such as between the thighs. List three other places they may develop on obese patients.

   1. _____

   2. _____

   3. _____

6. There are four stages of skin breakdown. Read each description below and write which stage it refers to.

   1. The layers of the skin have been destroyed and a deep crater has formed.

   _____

   2. The skin is reddened with blister-like lesions.

   _____

   3. The ulcer has eroded skin and other tissues.

   _____

   4. The skin is red and hot over an elbow.

   _____

7. You and a nurse will be working together to treat a patient with a decubitus ulcer. What will each of you do?

   _____

   _____

8. You notice that the patient's ulcer seems to be getting larger. What should you do?

   _____

9. There are many actions you can take while performing daily tasks to help prevent decubitus ulcers. After each routine task below, describe what you could do to prevent skin breakdown. The first one has been done for you.

   1. After a bath: Pat skin dry instead of rubbing it.

   2. When dressing a patient:

   _____

   3. During a back rub:

   _____

   4. When making a bed:

   _____

5. When changing an incontinent brief:

_____

6. When patients eat:

_____

Signature   **Date**

Chapter 15 • Learning Activities

MediaLink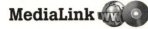

Additional free, interactive resources for this chapter can be found on the Student CD-ROM accompanying this book and on the Companion Website at **www.prenhall.com/pulliam**. Click on Chapter 15 to select activities for this chapter.

CD-ROM	**Companion Website**	
Audio Glossary	Audio Glossary	Matching
Certification Exam Review	Certification Exam Review	Study Tips
Animations/Videos:	Case Studies	MediaLink
Serving Food; Feeding a Dependent Patient	Challenge Your Knowledge	

Nutrition

1. Listed below is one reason why good nutrition is important for all people. What are three other reasons?

   1. It promotes physical and mental health.

   2. _____

   3. _____

   4. _____

2. From which food group do you need the most servings each day?

   _____

3. Which food group includes foods high in calories but low in nutrients?

   _____

4. Read the statements below and write which major nutrient each describes.

   1. These provide the most concentrated form of energy.

   _____

   2. These are essential for the growth and repair of tissues.

   _____

   3. These are chemicals that build body tissues and regulate body fluids.

   _____

   4. These provide the greatest amount of energy.

   _____

5. After the foods listed below, write which nutrient or nutrients each supplies.

1. Fish: _____

2. Fruits: _____

3. Breads: _____

4. Butter: _____

6. What are two of the reasons why people need water to maintain their health?

1. _____

2. _____

7. What is one way in which therapeutic diets differ from general diets?

_____

8. What type of therapeutic diet might a patient be on right after surgery?

_____

9. You serve a tray to a patient who is visually impaired. How can you assist her?

_____

_____

_____

10. When you serve food to a patient, at what time is it all right for you to leave her room?

_____

11. While feeding a dependent patient, you notice that he seems embarrassed that he can't feed himself. What should you do?

_____

12. If a physician gives a special fluid order of NPO, what should you do?

_____

13. What is a fluid imbalance?

_____

14. Listed below is one possible cause of dehydration. What are two other causes?

1. Insufficient intake.

2. _____

3. _____

15. Mrs. Jones has been placed on a clear liquid diet. Which of the following could be on her tray: tea, coffee, Sprite, apple juice, a popsicle, ice cream, yogurt, chicken broth, gelatin?

_____

16. Convert the following fluids from ounces to cubic centimeters using the formula 1 ounce equals 30 cc (cubic centimeters).

1. 4 ounces juice   = _____ cubic centimeters

2. 2.5 ounces soup = _____ cubic centimeters

3. 16 ounces water = _____ cubic centimeters

17. A patient has 8 ounces of tea on his tray before he eats his meal. After his meal, he has 3 ounces left. How many ounces did he drink? Using the formula in question 16, how many cubic centimeters was his input?

_____

18. When you observe bottles or bags on IVs, what are two of the problems you would have to alert the nurse to?

_____

_____

19. You have a patient with a nasogastric tube. What will you look for?

_____

_____

20. What procedure is never performed on an arm being used for an IV?

_____

_____
Signature   **Date**

MediaLink

Additional free, interactive resources for this chapter can be found on the Student CD-ROM accompanying this book and on the Companion Website at **www.prenhall.com/pulliam**. Click on Chapter 16 to select activities for this chapter.

CD-ROM	Companion Website	
Audio Glossary	Audio Glossary	Matching
Certification Exam Review	Certification Exam Review	Study Tips
Animations/Videos:	Case Studies	MediaLink
Nursing Assistant Responsibilities in Catheter Care	Challenge Your Knowledge	

Elimination Needs

1. Some of your patients urinate more frequently than others. Should you be concerned? Explain your answer.

_____

_____

2. A person's elimination frequency may be affected by diet. What are four other things that may affect frequency?

1. _____

2. _____

3. _____

4. _____

3. What are two of the ways you can help patients maintain normal elimination?

1. _____

2. _____

4. Describe normal urine.

_____

_____

5. A patient's feces are very watery. What should you do?

_____

6. What are some common causes of constipation?

_____

_____

7. How can you help a patient avoid constipation?

_____

_____

8. A patient of yours has diarrhea. What special care does she need?

_____

_____

_____

9. What should you do after removing soiled incontinent briefs?

_____

_____

10. A patient has trouble walking to the bathroom without assistance but is embarrassed to ask for help. How can you help him avoid having incontinent episodes?

_____

11. When you leave a patient who is sitting on a portable bedside commode, what do you need to do?

_____

12. A patient with a decubitus ulcer on her tailbone asks for a bedpan. What should you do?

_____

13. Listed below is one group of patients who may need more frequent perineal care than normal. Name three other groups.

1. Incontinent patients.

2. _____

3. _____

4. _____

14. Why is it important to rinse the perineum well when providing perineal care?

_____

15. What is the purpose of a urinary catheter?

_____

16. How can you help decrease the risk that patients with Foley catheters will get infections?

_____

_____

17. What do you need to observe and report when checking a patient's catheter?

_____

_____

18. Why does the drainage bag need to be kept below the level of the patient's bladder?

_____

19. When you empty a catheter drainage bag, what three things do you need to observe or check for?

1. _____

2. _____

3. _____

20. When you provide catheter care, what do you clean first? What do you clean next?

_____

_____

21. While providing catheter care to a patient, you find a disconnected tube. What should you do?

_____

Signature   **Date**

Chapter 17 • Learning Activities

MediaLink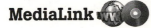

Additional free, interactive resources for this chapter can be found on the Student CD-ROM accompanying this book and on the Companion Website at **www.prenhall.com/pulliam**. Click on Chapter 17 to select activities for this chapter.

CD-ROM
Audio Glossary
Certification Exam Review
Animations/Videos:
*Guidelines for
Collecting Specimens*

Companion Website
Audio Glossary
Certification Exam Review
Case Studies
Challenge Your Knowledge

Matching
Study Tips
MediaLink

Specimen Collection and Testing

1. What does a physician use specimen test results for?

    1. _____
    2. _____
    3. _____

2. Who can draw blood specimens?

    _____

3. What are the three types of specimens nursing assistants may collect?

    1. _____
    2. _____
    3. _____

4. When you send a specimen to the laboratory, what must accompany it?

    _____

5. What information must be listed on a laboratory requisition slip?

    _____

6. Listed below is one item you need to fill out on a specimen label. What are four others?

    1. The patient's name.
    2. _____
    3. _____
    4. _____
    5. _____

7. While collecting a stool specimen, the patient contaminated it with urine. What should you do?

_____

_____

8. Listed below are descriptions of the four types of urine specimens: routine; midstream, clean-catch; 24-hour; fresh-fractional. After each one, write which type of specimen each describes.

   1. The patient urinates and then 30 minutes later the specimen is collected.

   _____

   2. The specimen is collected when the patient is admitted.

   _____

   3. A patient's urine is collected and saved for 24 hours.

   _____

   4. The urine specimen isn't contaminated by anything outside of the patient's body.

   _____

9. Why do you throw away the first amount the patient urinates when you collect a 24-hour urine specimen?

_____

_____

10. When can't a nursing assistant collect a routine urine specimen?

_____

_____

11. What does it mean if a physician orders a warm stool specimen?

_____

_____

12. What is the difference between sputum and saliva?

_____

_____

13. You need to collect a patient's sputum specimen. What time of day should you do it? Explain your answer.

_____

_____

_____
Signature   **Date**

Chapter 18 • Learning Activities

MediaLink

Additional free, interactive resources for this chapter can be found on the Student CD-ROM accompanying this book and on the Companion Website at **www.prenhall.com/ pulliam**. Click on Chapter 18 to select activities for this chapter.

CD-ROM	Companion Website	
Audio Glossary	Audio Glossary	Matching
Certification Exam Review	Certification Exam Review	Study Tips
Animations/Videos:	Case Studies	MediaLink
AM Care	Challenge Your Knowledge	

AM and PM Care

1. A patient has not slept well in nearly a week. How can this factor affect his recovery from his illness?

   _____

   _____

2. How much sleep does the *average* adult need per night?

   _____

3. What are two factors that influence the amount of sleep needed by people?

   1. _____

   2. _____

4. A patient complains of not being able to get enough sleep in the hospital. What symptoms should you look for in this patient that would indicate sleep deprivation?

   1. _____

   2. _____

   3. _____

   4. _____

5. How can you help patients get the rest and sleep they need?

_____

_____

_____

6. You have to enter the room of sleeping patients. What can you do to show consideration and not wake them?

_____

_____

_____

7. The following paragraph describes patient care in a health care facility throughout the day. Fill in the blanks with the appropriate term or phrase.

Nursing assistants meet the needs of patients in health care facilities

24 hours a day. Routine care that is administered when the patient

first wakes up is called (1) _____ or (2) _____ care.

Routine care that is administered before the patient goes to sleep

is called (3) _____ or (4) _____ care. Some health care

facilities use the term *HS care* instead of (5) _____. The

HS stands for the words (6) _____.

8. What is the best way to awaken patients?

_____

9. When should a patient *not* be awakened early for AM care?

_____

_____

10. During AM care, you normally assist patients with oral hygiene. What should you do if a newly admitted patient refuses to brush his teeth until after breakfast?

_____

_____

11. Your rotation shift involves giving AM care. What are some of the tasks you may need to perform as part of this procedure? One task has already been listed for you.

1. Offering a bedpan or urinal to patients or assisting patients with using the bathroom.

2. _____

3. _____

4. _____

5. _____

6. _____

7. _____

12. At bedtime a patient complains of tenseness and inability to fall asleep. What should you do to help him?

1. _____

2. _____

_____

Signature   **Date**

MediaLink

Additional free, interactive resources for this chapter can be found on the Student CD-ROM accompanying this book and on the Companion Website at **www.prenhall.com/pulliam**. Click on Chapter 19 to select activities for this chapter.

CD-ROM	Companion Website	
Audio Glossary	Audio Glossary	Matching
Certification Exam Review	Certification Exam Review	Study Tips
Animations/Videos:	Case Studies	MediaLink
Range-of-Motion Exercises	Challenge Your Knowledge	

Restorative Care and Rehabilitation

1. A woman is concerned about her husband's recovery from a stroke. The patient's physician mentioned *restorative care*. The woman asks you what this term means. What should you tell her?

   _____

   _____

   _____

2. A patient in your care is paralyzed from the waist down as a result of a diving accident. She wants to know what the term *rehabilitation* means. What should you tell her?

   _____

   _____

3. This same paralyzed patient wants to know which hospital personnel will be involved in helping her regain mobility and speech. What can you tell her about the following three members of the interdisciplinary team who teach patients to regain activities of daily living (ADL)?

   1. Occupational therapist: _____

   _____

   2. Physical therapist: _____

   _____

   3. Speech therapist: _____

   _____

4. A disabled person in your care needs to get dressed for physical therapy. One task you can perform to assist him is listed below. What are four others?

1. Provide privacy by pulling the curtain around the bed.

2. _____

3. _____

4. _____

5. _____

5. Various devices help patients who have impaired or missing body parts. The following paragraphs discuss these devices. Fill in the blanks with the appropriate term or phrase.

Supportive devices include those for walking or ambulating. Three examples of these devices are walkers, (1) _____, and (2) _____. Patients who cannot walk can use a (3) _____ or motorized chair. When a patient has a problem with balance, a (4) _____ should be used for ambulation activities. Artificial body parts, or (5) _____, help patients perform daily tasks and improve their self-image. Artificial supports, or (6) _____, are used when a body part is still present but is injured or impaired. (7) _____ are artificial supports that support a weak body part or hold a body part in position.

6. A patient in your care is undergoing bowel retraining. What time of the day is a good time to encourage this patient to defecate? Why?

_____

_____

7. As a nursing assistant, what guidelines should you follow in the bowel and bladder retraining of a patient?

1. _____

2. _____

3. _____

8. Range-of-motion exercises can be performed in bed. Below are two benefits of such exercises. List four other benefits of range-of-motion exercises.

1. They help to keep muscles strong and in good tone.

2. They help to promote blood circulation.

3. _____

4. _____

5. _____

6. _____

9. The following paragraph discusses the three types of range-of-motion exercises. Fill in the blanks with the terms that describe these exercises.

A nursing assistant's role in range-of-motion exercises varies according to the patient's abilities and the physician's orders. In (1) _____ range-of-motion exercises, the nursing assistant moves the patient's limbs through the exercises. Another type of range-of-motion exercise, (2) _____, involves the patient doing much of the exercise and then the nursing assistant helping with the rest. The third kind of range-of-motion exercise is called (3) _____. In this type of range of motion, the patient does the exercises without the help of the nursing assistant.

10. Below are photos showing various types of movement that occur when performing range-of-motion exercises. Study the photos, then write the type of movement each shows on the lines provided.

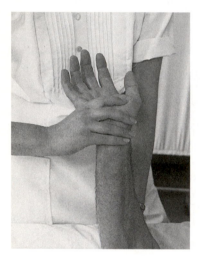 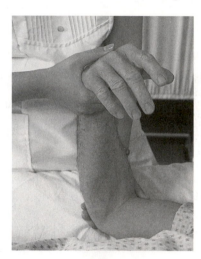 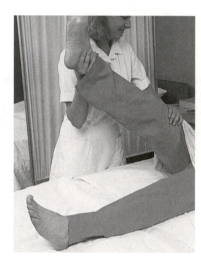

_____   _____   _____

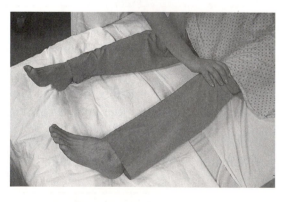

_____

_____

Signature   **Date**

Chapter 20 • Learning Activities

MediaLink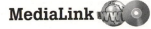

Additional free, interactive resources for this chapter can be found on the Student CD-ROM accompanying this book and on the Companion Website at **www.prenhall.com/pulliam**. Click on Chapter 20 to select activities for this chapter.

CD-ROM	Companion Website	
Audio Glossary	Audio Glossary	Matching
Certification Exam Review	Certification Exam Review	Study Tips
Animations/Videos:	Case Studies	MediaLink
Affects of Heat and Cold Treatments	Challenge Your Knowledge	

Additional Patient Care Procedures

1. A patient pulled a calf muscle yesterday. He complains that it is aching today. Would a physician order a heat treatment or a cold treatment for this patient? Why?

   _____

2. Would a physician usually order a heat or cold treatment for a patient with a freshly sprained ankle? Why?

   _____

   _____

3. A patient asks for a heat treatment for her aching back. What should you do?

   _____

   _____

4. A patient has been receiving cold treatments. You notice that the patient's skin looks blue, especially around the lips. What condition do you think he has?

   _____

   _____

   _____

5. The following paragraphs describe the variety of cold and heat treatments available to patients. Fill in each blank with the appropriate term or phrase.

Dry cold treatments should be used no more than (1) _____ minutes at a time. The basic cold treatment is the (2) _____, which is filled with ice chips or crushed ice. A special kind of cold treatment applied to the patient's neck is called an (3) _____.

There are two types of dry heat treatments. One, the (4) _____, has a special bulb and flexible neck so that heat can be directed at body parts from various distances. The other type of heat treatment, the (5) _____, differs from an electric heating pad because it has tubes filled with water inside the pad instead of wire coils.

6. What are three precautions that should be taken when using heat lamps?

   1. _____

   2. _____

   3. _____

7. For what reasons are sitz baths used? How often should you check a patient in a sitz bath?

   _____

   _____

   _____

8. Who can conduct a physical examination of a patient?

   _____

9. Nursing assistants have various responsibilities before, during, and after physical examinations. List three duties a nursing assistant should perform *before* the physical examination.

   1. _____

   2. _____

   3. _____

10. List three duties a nursing assistant should perform *during* the physical examination.

   1. _____

   2. _____

   3. _____

11. List three duties a nursing assistant should perform *after* the physical examination.

1. _____

2. _____

3. _____

12. During a physical examination, the physician tells you that she needs to examine the patient's eyes and ears. What two instruments would you get for the physician so that she could examine the patient's eyes and ears?

_____

_____

13. What type of enema is generally ordered by a physician for a patient with constipation?

_____

14. A physician has ordered a Harris flush for a patient. How would you describe this enema to the patient?

_____

_____

_____

_____

15. How long after a meal should you wait to give a patient an enema? How long should a patient retain, or hold, the fluid during an enema?

_____

_____

16. Your supervisor tells you to observe the results after you give a patient an enema. What does he mean?

_____

_____

_____

_____

_____   _____

Signature   **Date**

MediaLink

Additional free, interactive resources for this chapter can be found on the Student CD-ROM accompanying this book and on the Companion Website at **www.prenhall.com/pulliam**. Click on Chapter 21 to select activities for this chapter.

CD-ROM	**Companion Website**	
Audio Glossary	Audio Glossary	Matching
Certification Exam Review	Certification Exam Review	Study Tips
Animations/Videos:	Case Studies	MediaLink
Observations During Postoperative Care	Challenge Your Knowledge	

Preoperative and Postoperative Care

1. Many patients view surgery as a stressful experience. Listed below are two tasks you can perform to help patients undergoing surgery feel more relaxed. What are three more?

   1. Perform your work efficiently.

   2. Listen to the patient's fears and concerns.

   3. _____

   4. _____

   5. _____

2. Why are most surgery patients admitted on the morning of their operation rather than on the previous evening, as done in the past?

   _____

   _____

3. If a patient sneezes, sniffles, or coughs before surgery, why should it be reported to a supervisor?

   _____

   _____

   _____

4. A preoperative checklist ensures that a patient has been properly prepared for surgery. Fill in the following chart to create a checklist of preoperative care procedures a nursing assistant should perform on the morning of a patient's surgery.

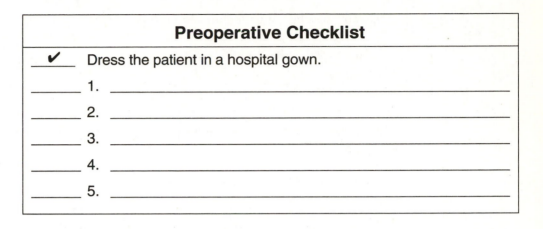

Preoperative Checklist

✔	Dress the patient in a hospital gown.
___ 1.	_____
___ 2.	_____
___ 3.	_____
___ 4.	_____
___ 5.	_____

5. A patient being prepared for surgery hears that a depilatory will be used on him. He asks what that means. What should you tell him?

_____

_____

6. What precaution must be taken before a depilatory is applied?

_____

7. Special medications are given to patients to block pain and relax muscles during surgery. The following paragraph describes these medications. Fill in the blanks with the appropriate term or phrase.

The name for special medications administered to patients to block pain and relax muscles during surgery is (1) _____. These medications can be administered four ways: (2) _____, (3) _____, (4) _____, and as an inhalant. A medication that blocks the brain from receiving pain is called a (5) _____. With use of this type of medication, a patient is not awake during surgery. Another type of medication used in surgery, a (6) _____, blocks only the area to be operated on from receiving pain. In this case, the patient is awake during surgery. A (7) _____ is administered at the spinal cord and usually causes loss of feeling from the navel to the feet. Special care must be taken in administering all these medications.

8. Anesthetics may cause a patient to feel nauseous and to vomit. What are two dangers that vomited material might cause if it is aspirated?

    1. _____

    2. _____

9. You are checking the intravenous tube of a postoperative patient. You notice that the clamp on the tube is loose and that the rate of infusion seems to have increased. What should you do?

    _____

    _____

10. What are two types of exercise that can help patients avoid complications after surgery?

    1. _____

    2. _____

11. What are binders and where are they usually applied?

    _____

    _____

12. What is used to prevent or treat phlebitis?

    _____

    _____

13. One day after surgery, a patient is ready for initial ambulation. What procedure should be practiced before ambulation occurs?

    _____

14. What are three benefits of dangling?

    1. _____

    2. _____

    3. _____

Signature   **Date**

MediaLink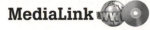

Additional free, interactive resources for this chapter can be found on the Student CD-ROM accompanying this book and on the Companion Website at **www.prenhall.com/pulliam**. Click on Chapter 22 to select activities for this chapter.

CD-ROM	**Companion Website**	
Audio Glossary	Audio Glossary	Matching
Certification Exam Review	Certification Exam Review	Study Tips
	Case Studies	MediaLink
	Challenge Your Knowledge	

Subacute Care

1. What characteristics or conditions do patients who are admitted to subacute care facilities have?

   1. _____
   2. _____
   3. _____

2. Listed below is one service available to subacute care patients. What are three others?

   1. Pharmaceutical services.
   2. _____
   3. _____
   4. _____

3. What is the average length of stay for a transitional subacute patient?

   _____

4. Name three requirements a patient must meet to be admitted to a subacute care facility.

   1. _____
   2. _____
   3. _____

5. List two goals for a transitional subacute care patient.

   1. _____
   2. _____

6. What are two important factors to be considered when charting for subacute patients?

    1. _____

    2. _____

7. List four kinds of invasive equipment that a subacute patient might be using.

    1. _____

    2. _____

    3. _____

    4. _____

8. List three patient needs that subacute care is designed to meet.

    1. _____

    2. _____

    3. _____

9. Why must nursing assistants have good team and organizational skills?

_____

_____

_____

10. List three signs of a possible problem with a patient's wound.

    1. _____

    2. _____

    3. _____

11. Describe a situation in which your ability to be flexible with your planned patient care would work to the benefit of the whole team and the patient.

_____

_____

_____

_____

_____

12. What kind of thermometer would you not use for a disoriented patient?

_____

_____

_____
Signature   **Date**

Chapter 23 • Learning Activities

MediaLink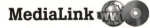

Additional free, interactive resources for this chapter can be found on the Student CD-ROM accompanying this book and on the Companion Website at **www.prenhall.com/pulliam**. Click on Chapter 23 to select activities for this chapter.

CD-ROM
Audio Glossary
Certification Exam Review
Animations/Videos:
  Communicating with
  Cognitively Impaired
  Residents

Companion Website
Audio Glossary
Certification Exam Review
Case Studies
Challenge Your Knowledge

Matching
Study Tips
MediaLink

Special Skills in Long-Term Care

1. What types of people are admitted to long-term care facilities as residents?

   1. _____

   2. _____

   3. _____

2. Listed below is one task a nursing assistant can perform to help residents and their families during a nursing home adjustment period. What are four others?

   1. Orient the resident and family members.

   2. _____

   3. _____

   4. _____

   5. _____

3. An elderly patient who is usually cooperative tells you she wants to stay in her nightgown and robe today. What should you do?

   _____

   _____

4. Every weekend a resident's son visits his mother at the facility and criticizes the way you care for his mother. What should you do?

   _____

   _____

5. At least once a week at mealtime, an elderly man masturbates before eating. This makes the other residents uncomfortable. What should you do?

_____

_____

_____

6. Upon entering the room of a disabled resident, you discover the resident and her spouse engaging in sexual activity. What should you do?

_____

7. What are three ways in which you can help residents of long-term care facilities express their sexuality?

1. _____

2. _____

3. _____

8. Elderly people must make various emotional and social adjustments in adapting to old age. For example, they must adjust to an altered body image. List three other emotional or social adjustments they may have to make.

1. _____

2. _____

3. _____

9. A disabled resident who is usually cheerful and upbeat has been acting angry and violent all week. What should you do? Why?

_____

_____

10. Listed below is one way nursing assistants can help residents meet spiritual needs. What are two other ways they can assist in this task?

1. Read religious literature to residents upon request.

2. _____

3. _____

11. Recreational activities break daily routines and make facility living more pleasant. How can nursing assistants help residents meet their recreational needs?

_____

_____

_____

_____

12. Why are elderly people more prone to choking than younger people?

_____

13. Loss of memory has long been a concern of elderly people. The following paragraph discusses this topic. Fill in the blanks with the appropriate term or phrase.

(1) _____ refers to a diminished ability to think and remember.

Despite popular belief, mental deterioration is not a normal

process of aging. Mental deterioration is often caused by disease.

The chronic, organic decline of mental ability is (2) _____.

Three common causes of this condition are (3) _____,

(4) _____, and Huntington's disease. The condition of memory

deterioration that is responsible for about half of dementias is

(5) _____. One early sign of this disease is (6) _____. As

the disease progresses, more serious symptoms follow.

14. What are the four factors that may trigger difficult behavior in residents with dementia?

1. _____

2. _____

3. _____

4. _____

15. During dinner, a resident becomes agitated and almost violent. What should you do?

_____

_____

_____

16. What is validation therapy and how does it help make mental deterioration less damaging to a person's self-esteem?

_____

_____

_____   _____
Signature   Date

MediaLink

Additional free, interactive resources for this chapter can be found on the Student CD-ROM accompanying this book and on the Companion Website at **www.prenhall.com/pulliam**. Click on Chapter 24 to select activities for this chapter.

CD-ROM	**Companion Website**	
Audio Glossary	Audio Glossary	Matching
Certification Exam Review	Certification Exam Review	Study Tips
Animations/Videos:	Case Studies	MediaLink
Stages of Dying	Challenge Your Knowledge	

Death and Dying

1. The elderly patient you are caring for is telling you that he doesn't believe his diagnosis of colon cancer. "Not me," says this terminally ill patient. "I'm as healthy as a horse!" How should you respond?

   _____

   _____

2. Throwing a book to the floor, a terminally ill teenager shouts, "Why me?" He then turns to his mother and says, "I'm too young to die!" According to Kübler-Ross, in what stage of dying is this patient?

   _____

3. What are four ways that your attitude about death can affect your care of a dying patient?

   1. _____

   2. _____

   3. _____

   4. _____

4. How can you help terminally ill patients prepare spiritually for death?

   _____

   _____

5. Spiritual preparation of dying patients is important. List two Roman Catholic customs that a dying patient of this faith may want you to follow.

1. _____

2. _____

6. A Jewish patient has died. Should you touch the body? Explain your answer.

_____

_____

7. Visitors' hours ended over a half hour ago. When you enter the room of a terminally ill patient, her three children are still by her bed. What should you do? Why?

_____

_____

8. What is your primary goal in caring for a dying patient?

_____

9. Why should you speak to an unconscious patient? How should you speak?

_____

_____

_____

10. You notice that a dying patient is breathing heavily through his mouth. Upon closer inspection, you discover that his mouth is dry and irritated. How should you treat this condition?

_____

_____

11. What are three procedures you could perform to make breathing easier for a dying patient?

1. _____

2. _____

3. _____

12. Why do some dying patients have anal and urinary incontinence?

_____

_____

13. Rather than solids and liquids, what types of food may be easier for a dying patient to handle?

_____

14. What does a DNR or "no code" order tell the health care team about a dying patient?

_____

_____

15. Who writes a DNR order?

_____

16. A terminally ill patient asks you what types of care can be prohibited in an advance directive. One is listed below. What are three others?

1. Resuscitation

2. _____

3. _____

4. _____

17. An AIDS patient asks you what is meant by the term _hospice care_. What should you tell him?

_____

_____

_____

_____

_____

18. After death, the body continues to change. Two changes are listed below. What are four other changes that occur after death?

1. Permanently fixed and dilated pupils.

2. Gradual loss of body heat.

3. _____

4. _____

5. _____

6. _____

19. What is postmortem care? When should you begin it?

_____

_____

_____

Signature   **Date**

Chapter 1 • Quiz

Introduction to Health Care

Read each statement carefully. Then circle the letter of the best answer for each item.

1. An illness for which there is no known cure is called:

   (A) acute.
   (B) abnormal.
   (C) psychiatric.
   (D) chronic.

2. Medicare and Medicaid payments are based on:

   (A) the length of the patient's treatment.
   (B) the patient's annual salary.
   (C) the type of illness or condition treated.
   (D) an annual lottery.

3. Which of the following is *not* a common purpose of health care facilities?

   (A) To provide treatment for diseases
   (B) To improve health insurance
   (C) To rehabilitate persons who have injuries
   (D) To promote medical research

4. Most acute care hospital stays are:

   (A) less than 2 days.
   (B) a few days or weeks.
   (C) several months.
   (D) for the rest of the patient's life.

5. Long-term care facilities provide health care for:

   (A) patients who cannot afford to go to a hospital.
   (B) veterans and government workers.
   (C) people who are unable to care for themselves.
   (D) infants and children.

6. A nursing assistant usually reports to a team leader. In some facilities, the team leader might be called a(n):

   (A) administrator.
   (B) physician.
   (C) charge nurse.
   (D) resident.

7. An interdisciplinary team may be made up of:

(A) nurses and nursing assistants.
(B) therapists to include physical therapy, occupational therapy, and speech therapy.
(C) patients and doctors.
(D) all of the above.

8. A Kardex file is used to provide a central source of information about:

(A) facility employees.
(B) each patient.
(C) physicians.
(D) illnesses and their treatment.

9. The care plan is created and followed by:

(A) a nursing assistant.
(B) a registered nurse.
(C) the interdisciplinary team.
(D) the patient.

10. What is a diagnosis?

(A) An identification of the cause and nature of the patient's problems
(B) A list of short-term and long-term goals for the patient
(C) A list of the medications given to a patient
(D) A patient's history of illness

11. Gloria is a registered nurse. She is in charge of planning and implementing all of the care for six patients on her hospital floor. This is an example of nursing care organization called:

(A) functional nursing.
(B) primary nursing.
(C) team nursing.
(D) interdisciplinary nursing.

12. Mr. Valdez is recovering from surgery. After a 2-week hospital stay, he returns to his home. Care is provided by a business that sends workers to his home. This type of business is an example of:

(A) a home health agency.
(B) a nursing home.
(C) a rehabilitation center.
(D) a psychiatric hospital.

_____

Signature   **Date**

Chapter 2 • Quiz

The Nursing Assistant

Read each statement carefully. Then circle the letter of the best answer for each item.

1. The term *scope of practice* refers to all of the duties that a nursing assistant is:

   (A) legally permitted to perform.
   (B) expected to perform each day.
   (C) can perform in an emergency.
   (D) required to perform by law.

2. Nursing assistants are *not* permitted to:

   (A) transport patients from one area of the facility to another.
   (B) help patients with personal needs.
   (C) take a patient's vital signs.
   (D) administer medications.

3. According to the "Patient's Bill of Rights," a patient has the right to:

   (A) leave the facility without paying for care.
   (B) a private hospital room.
   (C) refuse treatment.
   (D) home health care.

4. Which of the following actions is an example of negligence?

   (A) A physician does not renew a patient's medication order.
   (B) A nursing assistant does not reposition a bed-confined patient as instructed.
   (C) A registered nurse performs sterile procedures.
   (D) A nursing assistant refuses to discuss a patient's diagnosis with a visitor.

5. A nursing assistant can be guilty of false imprisonment if she:

   (A) restrains a patient without proper authority.
   (B) closes a patient's door without asking permission.
   (C) restricts the number of visitors according to facility policy.
   (D) yells at or threatens a patient.

6. Nursing assistants should:

   (A) report and document changes in a patient's condition.
   (B) share their personal problems openly with coworkers.
   (C) avoid contact with their supervisors.
   (D) leave when work is finished, regardless of what time it is.

7. Who establishes priorities when planning work assignments?

   (A) The nursing assistant
   (B) The interdisciplinary team
   (C) The nurse in charge or team leader
   (D) The patient

8. To help manage stress, it is wise for health care workers to:

   (A) limit their sleep to 6 hours a night.
   (B) reduce their calorie intake.
   (C) exercise regularly.
   (D) limit leisure activities.

9. Standard precautions are intended to prevent workers from:

   (A) being negligent.
   (B) being exposed to potentially dangerous body fluids.
   (C) working outside of their scope of practice.
   (D) experiencing burnout.

10. The term *liable* means:

    (A) unnecessary.
    (B) possibly harmful.
    (C) negligent.
    (D) legally responsible.

11. A nursing assistant is responsible for:

    (A) answering a patient's letters and phone calls.
    (B) keeping a patient's personal information confidential.
    (C) filing a patient's complaints with hospital administration.
    (D) recommending medications and treatments.

12. A nursing assistant belittles a patient by telling her that she is overreacting to her condition. This is an example of:

    (A) physical abuse.
    (B) false imprisonment.
    (C) negligence.
    (D) psychological abuse.

_____

Signature   **Date**

Chapter 3 • Quiz

Communication and Interpersonal Skills

Read each statement carefully. Then circle the letter of the best answer for each item.

1. Which of the following is an example of verbal communication?

    (A) The writing on a patient's chart
    (B) Tone of voice
    (C) Body language
    (D) Facial expressions

2. To be a good listener, you should avoid:

    (A) showing interest and concern.
    (B) direct eye contact.
    (C) interrupting the speaker.
    (D) nonverbal communication.

3. Which of the following statements might imply that the patient's feelings are unimportant?

    (A) "Don't worry. Everything will be okay."
    (B) "I know that this is difficult for you."
    (C) "You are looking very well today."
    (D) "Please tell me if there's anything I can do for you."

4. When a patient uses a call signal, you should:

    (A) ask your supervisor what to do.
    (B) go at once to the patient's room.
    (C) wait to see if another worker is going to respond first.
    (D) finish your assigned duties before responding to the patient.

5. Which of the following is an example of a subjective observation?

    (A) You notice that a patient has developed a rash.
    (B) You hear a patient coughing throughout the night.
    (C) You find that a patient has a fever.
    (D) You notice that a patient is less talkative than usual.

6. Chart entries should always:

    (A) be made in pencil.
    (B) include the date and time.
    (C) use ditto marks to indicate repeated information.
    (D) be written at the end of your shift.

7. You should immediately contact your supervisor if you notice that a patient is:

   (A) eating less than usual.
   (B) having difficulty breathing.
   (C) coughing.
   (D) feeling better.

8. When studying medical terminology, which part of the word gives the word's primary meaning?

   (A) The word root
   (B) The prefix
   (C) The tense
   (D) The suffix

9. A patient's chart is primarily used to:

   (A) keep track of billing information.
   (B) indicate each worker's scope of practice.
   (C) help the health care team communicate with one another.
   (D) provide evidence of negligence or malpractice.

10. Hal is a nursing assistant. His patient is Ms. Baker. She wants to stop taking one of her medications. She tells Hal, who passes the information on to the charge nurse. The charge nurse asks Hal about Ms. Baker's concern. In this situation, the feedback is:

    (A) Ms. Baker's complaint.
    (B) Hal's careful attention to Ms. Baker's condition.
    (C) the charge nurse's questions about the situation.
    (D) the medication.

11. Ms. Brown is filling in a patient's chart. She makes a mistake. What should she do?

    (A) Make a new chart with the correct information.
    (B) Ask her supervisor to make the chart entry.
    (C) Cross out the mistake, write your initials above it, and then write the correct information.
    (D) Leave the mistake unchanged, but include the correct information in the chart as well.

12. When communicating over the telephone, you should:

    (A) not take messages unless they are urgent.
    (B) speak as quickly as possible to be efficient.
    (C) identify yourself when you answer.
    (D) use nonverbal communication to help make your message clear.

_____

Signature   **Date**

Relating to Your Patients

Read each statement carefully. Then circle the letter of the best answer for each item.

1. According to Abraham Maslow, which category of human need must be satisfied before any other?

   (A) Self-actualization
   (B) Belongingness and love
   (C) Safety and security
   (D) Physiological

2. To help a patient adjust to an illness, you should:

   (A) tell the patient not to feel sad.
   (B) assure the patient that everything will be all right.
   (C) allow the patient to express feelings and concerns.
   (D) try to limit the number of decisions the patient has to make.

3. What should you do if a patient starts to cry?

   (A) Say "Don't worry, you're going to be fine."
   (B) Ask the patient to stop crying because it upsets others.
   (C) Soothe the patient but let the patient know it is all right to cry.
   (D) Ignore the emotion to avoid embarrassing the patient.

4. If a patient becomes physically threatening, the first thing you should do is:

   (A) restrain the patient.
   (B) back away.
   (C) lock the patient in a room.
   (D) call the security department of your facility.

5. Loss of interest in eating is often a sign of:

   (A) aggressive behavior.
   (B) demanding behavior.
   (C) self-centered behavior.
   (D) depression.

6. You should always avoid:

   (A) shouting at patients.
   (B) direct eye contact with patients.
   (C) using physical restraints on patients.
   (D) the people who come to visit a patient.

7. When caring for people from different cultures, you should try to:

    (A) avoid talking to them.
    (B) pretend that the cultural differences do not exist.
    (C) encourage them to change their beliefs while in your facility.
    (D) understand and respect their special needs.

8. If a patient is unconscious, you should assume that the patient:

    (A) cannot hear anything you say.
    (B) can only hear words spoken very loudly.
    (C) can hear and understand you.
    (D) has no mental abilities.

9. Karen is working with Mr. Ahn, who lives in a long-term care facility. She encourages him to make his own decisions about what to do each day. She helps him with dressing and grooming, but lets him do as much as he can himself. These activities help provide for Mr. Ahn's need for:

    (A) self-esteem.
    (B) shelter.
    (C) security.
    (D) spirituality.

10. Marissa feels that one of her patients is strongly prejudiced against her. What should she do?

    (A) Avoid caring for that patient.
    (B) Confront the patient and argue for her rights.
    (C) Give that patient the same care she gives any other patient.
    (D) Refuse to care for the patient unless this attitude changes.

11. If a patient has a sight impairment, it is always a good idea to:

    (A) speak very slowly.
    (B) stand at least 3 feet away from the patient.
    (C) identify yourself when you enter the patient's room.
    (D) begin procedures without explaining what you will be doing.

12. Controlling the level of noise in a patient's room will help to provide for the need for:

    (A) food.
    (B) rest.
    (C) approval and acceptance.
    (D) respect and dignity.

_____

Signature   **Date**

Infection Control

Read each statement carefully. Then circle the letter of the best answer for each item.

1. What are pathogens?

   (A) Any living organisms that are too small to see with the eye
   (B) Living things that cause disease
   (C) The means by which diseases are transmitted
   (D) Any medications used to treat a disease

2. Most bacteria grow best at:

   (A) temperatures below the freezing point.
   (B) temperatures colder than body temperature.
   (C) body temperature.
   (D) temperatures higher than body temperature.

3. Pathogens are most likely to grow in places that are:

   (A) sterile.
   (B) antiseptic.
   (C) bright and dry.
   (D) moist and dark.

4. The organism that causes an infection is called the:

   (A) causative agent.
   (B) reservoir of the agent.
   (C) portal of entry.
   (D) susceptible host.

5. A bedpan that becomes contaminated by a patient's excretions is an example of a:

   (A) carrier.
   (B) portal of entry.
   (C) fomite.
   (D) pathogen.

6. If transmission of a disease involves an intermediate host such as a flea or mosquito, the transmission is called:

   (A) direct.
   (B) airborne.
   (C) indirect.
   (D) vector-borne.

7. A nosocomial infection is one that:

   (A) is acquired as a result of being in a health care facility.
   (B) is transmitted by infectious droplets.
   (C) cannot be transmitted from one person to another.
   (D) restricts the body's immune response.

8. In a health care facility, a set of linens is called clean only if it:

   (A) has been sterilized.
   (B) contains no microorganisms.
   (C) is not contaminated by pathogens.
   (D) has never been used before.

9. You should use standard precautions when:

   (A) a patient is known to be infectious.
   (B) a patient has a cognitive impairment.
   (C) treating elderly patients.
   (D) treating any patient.

10. To be certain that all microorganisms on an item have been killed, the item should be:

    (A) washed in hot water.
    (B) disinfected.
    (C) cleaned with strong detergents.
    (D) sterilized.

11. Transmission-based precautions are designed to:

    (A) prevent the spread of infection in a health care facility.
    (B) protect the patient from pathogens possibly carried by people entering the room.
    (C) disinfect a patient unit after the patient is discharged.
    (D) make standard precautions unnecessary.

12. Which of the following techniques does *not* promote medical asepsis?

    (A) Washing your hands before performing a procedure
    (B) Cleaning all reusable equipment immediately after use
    (C) Holding food trays away from your body
    (D) Sitting on a patient's bed

_____

Signature   **Date**

Environmental Safety, Accident Prevention, and Disaster Plans

Read each statement carefully. Then circle the letter of the best answer for each item.

1. To make sure you have the right patient before giving care:

   (A) ask another nursing assistant.
   (B) ask the patient his or her name.
   (C) check the patient's identification bracelet.
   (D) check the patient's chart or nursing care plan.

2. Before you begin any procedure:

   (A) make sure you have the right patient.
   (B) take the patient's blood pressure.
   (C) raise the bed to its highest position.
   (D) help the patient sit up.

3. The most common type of accident in health care facilities is:

   (A) poisoning.
   (B) burns.
   (C) falls.
   (D) suffocation.

4. Elderly people are at particular risk for burns because they:

   (A) may be disoriented.
   (B) may be overmedicated.
   (C) may be slow to feel hot temperatures.
   (D) may not follow smoking rules.

5. If you can't read a medicine label:

   (A) put the medicine back where you got it.
   (B) ask a coworker what the medicine is.
   (C) throw the medicine away.
   (D) take the medicine to your supervisor right away.

6. When you use proper body mechanics, you:

   (A) keep your feet close together.
   (B) hold heavy objects close to your body.
   (C) bend from the waist.
   (D) twist at the waist.

7. Restraints are used to limit patients' movements:

   (A) when no other means can effectively protect them.
   (B) when you don't have time to check on them.
   (C) whenever patients act combative.
   (D) whenever you think they're necessary.

8. Studies show that restrained patients:

   (A) have as many accidents as unrestrained patients.
   (B) don't have any accidents.
   (C) have fewer accidents than unrestrained patients.
   (D) have twice as many accidents as unrestrained patients.

9. Which item below is *not* needed to start a fire?

   (A) Oxygen
   (B) Fuel
   (C) Heat
   (D) Electricity

10. A major cause of fire in health care facilities is:

    (A) improper use of oxygen.
    (B) smoking.
    (C) unsafe practices in kitchens.
    (D) arson.

11. If a fire starts, the first thing you need to do is:

    (A) contain the fire.
    (B) activate the alarm.
    (C) extinguish the fire.
    (D) remove the patients to safety.

12. During a disaster, your first priority is:

    (A) ensuring the safety of your patients.
    (B) helping your co-workers.
    (C) calling for outside assistance.
    (D) taking care of yourself.

_____

Signature   **Date**

Chapter 7 • Quiz

Emergency Situations

Read each statement carefully. Then circle the letter of the best answer for each item.

1. Which of the following situations is a life-threatening emergency?

   (A) A patient's pulse decreases.
   (B) A patient is in shock.
   (C) A patient refuses to eat.
   (D) A patient is withdrawn and depressed.

2. The first action you should take upon discovering an emergency situation is:

   (A) file an emergency procedures report.
   (B) ask the patient to recommend treatment.
   (C) assess the problem.
   (D) call or send for help.

3. What happens during cardiac arrest?

   (A) Heart function and circulation stop.
   (B) Respiration stops due to a blocked airway.
   (C) A patient has a grand mal seizure.
   (D) Pulse and respiration increase rapidly.

4. The notation *no code* or *DNR* on a patient's chart means that this patient:

   (A) is highly contagious.
   (B) should not be given any medications.
   (C) has medical allergies which must be considered before determining treatment.
   (D) should not be resuscitated in the event of cardiac or respiratory failure.

5. Which of the following is *not* a sign that a patient's heartbeat and breathing may have stopped?

   (A) The skin is hot.
   (B) The chest is not expanding.
   (C) The patient is unconscious.
   (D) The pupils in the eyes are enlarged.

6. A patient has no pulse. To restore circulation, you should use:

   (A) artificial or mouth-to-mouth breathing.
   (B) the Heimlich maneuver.
   (C) the finger sweep.
   (D) artificial breathing with chest compression.

7. What is the most common cause of choking in adults?

   (A) Vomiting
   (B) Coughing up blood
   (C) Blockage by a foreign object
   (D) Swallowing saliva

8. If a choking victim is coughing violently, you should:

   (A) try to get the patient to stop coughing.
   (B) allow the coughing to continue.
   (C) immediately begin the Heimlich maneuver.
   (D) use chest compression and artificial breathing.

9. The finger sweep is used to:

   (A) clear the blocked airway of an unconscious patient.
   (B) restore circulation.
   (C) reduce the possibility of injury during a seizure.
   (D) restrain patients during violent seizures.

10. If a patient is undergoing a seizure, it is most important to:

    (A) stop the seizure.
    (B) reduce the possibility of future seizures.
    (C) protect the patient from infection and disease.
    (D) protect the patient from physical injury.

11. When a patient is undergoing a seizure, you should:

    (A) use restraints to limit the patient's movements.
    (B) place a towel or blanket under the head.
    (C) tighten the patient's clothing, especially around the neck.
    (D) place an object in the mouth to prevent injury.

12. An unconscious patient has a blocked airway. She is lying on the ground but does not have a head, neck, or spine injury. The first thing you should do to open the airway is:

    (A) tilt the head forward, pushing the chin toward the chest.
    (B) lift the head off the ground and shake gently.
    (C) tilt the head backward and lift the chin.
    (D) shake the head gently from side to side.

_____

Signature   **Date**

Chapter 8 • Quiz

Body Systems and Common Diseases

Read each statement carefully. Then circle the letter of the best answer for each item.

1. Groups of tissues that perform one or more specific functions are called:

   (A) cells.
   (B) organs.
   (C) microorganisms.
   (D) systems.

2. A genetic disease is one that is:

   (A) inherited from the parents.
   (B) fatal.
   (C) an autoimmune disorder.
   (D) undetectable during early stages of growth and development.

3. HIV is transmitted:

   (A) through the exchange of body fluids.
   (B) through the air.
   (C) through food.
   (D) through infectious droplets in the air.

4. If a tumor is benign, it:

   (A) grows quickly.
   (B) spreads to other parts of the body.
   (C) does not invade surrounding tissue.
   (D) cannot be removed.

5. Chronic bronchitis is an inflammation of the air tubes in the lungs. It is a disorder of the:

   (A) circulatory system.
   (B) gastrointestinal system.
   (C) endocrine system.
   (D) respiratory system.

6. The leading causes of death in the United States are:

   (A) cardiovascular diseases.
   (B) cancers.
   (C) autoimmune disorders.
   (D) diseases of the nervous system.

7. Involuntary muscle contractions called peristalsis:

    (A) cause muscles to shorten.
    (B) make motion possible.
    (C) move food through the digestive system.
    (D) result in arthritis.

8. What is an ostomy?

    (A) A surgical procedure that provides an alternate route for wastes
    (B) A disorder of the urinary system
    (C) The removal of waste products from the blood by a hemodialysis machine
    (D) High blood sugar

9. Which of the following is a disease of the endocrine system?

    (A) Diabetes
    (B) Arthritis
    (C) Arteriosclerosis
    (D) Emphysema

10. In which body system does the skin function?

    (A) Musculoskeletal
    (B) Circulatory
    (C) Integumentary
    (D) Nervous

11. When caring for a patient with a newly applied leg cast, you should:

    (A) cover the cast with a light blanket or plastic sheet.
    (B) place the cast on a hard, level surface.
    (C) leave the patient in one position until the cast is dried.
    (D) support the entire length of the cast with pillows.

12. When caring for stroke patients, you should:

    (A) avoid talking to them.
    (B) encourage the patients to be as independent as possible.
    (C) expect the patients to feed and dress themselves.
    (D) make sure that the patients remain in one position throughout the day.

_____

Signature   **Date**

Chapter 9 • Quiz

Vital Signs

Read each statement carefully. Then circle the letter of the best answer for each item.

1. Which of the following is *not* one of the body's vital signs?

   (A) Blood pressure
   (B) Pulse
   (C) Respiration
   (D) Digestion

2. What are baseline measurements?

   (A) The lowest safe levels that vital signs can reach
   (B) A patient's vital signs when admitted to a facility
   (C) The normal vital sign measurements for adults
   (D) Measurements of height and weight

3. The least accurate method of measuring body temperature is:

   (A) oral measurement.
   (B) rectal measurement.
   (C) axillary measurement.
   (D) aural measurement.

4. When using a glass oral thermometer, you should:

   (A) always shake down the mercury before each use.
   (B) be careful to never shake the thermometer.
   (C) run the thermometer under very hot water immediately before use.
   (D) never leave the thermometer in the patient's mouth for more than 1 minute.

5. When washing a glass thermometer, you should use:

   (A) boiling water and detergent.
   (B) cold water and soap.
   (C) warm water and alcohol.
   (D) a clean, dry towel only.

6. Which of the following pulse rates is abnormal and should be reported to a supervisor?

   (A) 67 beats per minute
   (B) 74 beats per minute
   (C) 45 beats per minute
   (D) 88 beats per minute

7. The most common method of measuring pulse is to measure the:

   (A) radial pulse.
   (B) apical pulse.
   (C) respiratory rate.
   (D) blood pressure.

8. When you are measuring respiration, you should:

   (A) always tell the patient that you are measuring breathing.
   (B) not tell the patient that you are measuring breathing.
   (C) ask the patient to breathe as deeply as possible.
   (D) ask the patient to breathe as quickly as possible.

9. A sphygmomanometer is used to measure:

   (A) pulse.
   (B) body temperature.
   (C) blood pressure.
   (D) respiration.

10. When measuring a patient's blood pressure, you should:

    (A) take your reading immediately after the patient has been exercising.
    (B) apply the cuff over the patient's sleeve.
    (C) use the stethoscope to measure the apical pulse.
    (D) apply the cuff to the upper arm above the brachial artery.

11. Charles took a patient's temperature with an oral thermometer. He noticed that the reading was considerably outside the normal range and told his supervisor. Which of the following temperatures might the patient have measured?

    (A) 98.2°F
    (B) 97.9°F
    (C) 101.2°F
    (D) 99.1°F

12. Dyan measured a conscious patient's radial pulse. She placed her thumb on the patient's wrist and pressed gently. She measured the pulse she felt for 1 full minute. Why might her reading be inaccurate?

    (A) You should only take apical pulses for conscious patients.
    (B) You should measure the pulse for more than 1 minute.
    (C) You should not use your thumb to measure a pulse.
    (D) You should not press on the wrist when taking a pulse.

_____   _____
Signature   **Date**

Positioning, Moving, and Ambulation

Read each statement carefully. Then circle the letter of the best answer for each item.

1. If a patient's body is correctly aligned in bed, the spine should be:

   (A) slightly curved.
   (B) 6 inches above the mattress.
   (C) straight.
   (D) twisted to relieve pressure.

2. Shearing can be reduced by:

   (A) sliding patients whenever possible.
   (B) lifting or rolling patients.
   (C) discouraging ambulation.
   (D) changing a patient's diet.

3. A trochanter roll is used to:

   (A) keep a patient's hips and legs from turning out.
   (B) keep the mattress from sagging.
   (C) prevent ambulation.
   (D) move a helpless patient.

4. Bed-confined patients are turned regularly to avoid:

   (A) ambulation.
   (B) respiratory failure.
   (C) hypothermia.
   (D) skin breakdown.

5. When turning a patient, it is helpful if the patient:

   (A) remains as stiff as possible.
   (B) crosses his or her legs.
   (C) grips onto the side of the bed.
   (D) is restrained before beginning the procedure.

6. It is most likely that you would be asked to logroll a patient who has:

   (A) a respiratory illness.
   (B) a spinal-cord injury.
   (C) cardiovascular disease.
   (D) AIDS.

7. When a patient is sitting in a chair, his or her back should:

(A) not touch the back of the chair.
(B) be supported by the back of the chair.
(C) be curved forward.
(D) twist to one side.

8. Which of the following is not a mechanical aid used for ambulation?

(A) Cane
(B) Walker
(C) Gait belt
(D) Postural support

9. When assisting a patient to ambulate using a cane:

(A) the patient should use the cane to stand.
(B) the cane should be moved 2 to 4 inches ahead of the patient.
(C) the patient should hold the cane on the strong side of the body.
(D) the patient should hold the cane on the weak side of the body.

10. Mona is using a transfer belt to support a patient during transfer. Before beginning the procedure, she should make sure that the belt is:

(A) tight enough to impair breathing slightly.
(B) slack enough to allow her hand to fit inside.
(C) snug enough to allow only two fingers inside the belt.
(D) unbuckled.

11. What position is used for a patient who wishes to eat in bed?

(A) Fowler's
(B) Supine
(C) Prone
(D) Lateral

12. Which of the following is not a correct procedure to follow when caring for a falling patient?

(A) Hold a falling patient at arm's length.
(B) Lower the patient to the floor as gently as possible.
(C) Do not leave the patient.
(D) Slide the patient down one leg, sitting as you go.

_____

Signature   **Date**

Admission, Transfer, and Discharge

Read each statement carefully. Then circle the letter of the best answer for each item.

1. The set of procedures that marks a patient's entry into a health care facility is called:

   (A) transfer.
   (B) discharge.
   (C) admission.
   (D) long-term care.

2. A patient is moved from a semiprivate room to a private room. This is an example of:

   (A) an admission.
   (B) a discharge.
   (C) a restraint.
   (D) a transfer.

3. The main effect of DRGs (diagnosis-related groups) on health care is that patients under these plans:

   (A) are no longer guaranteed medical care.
   (B) may be discharged earlier than in the past.
   (C) no longer require home care.
   (D) have limited patients' rights.

4. Which of the following admission processes is *not* done by a nursing assistant?

   (A) Preparing the unit for the patient
   (B) Welcoming the patient
   (C) Diagnosing the patient
   (D) Gathering information about the patient

5. A patient's personal items such as eyeglasses and dentures should be:

   (A) sent home with family members.
   (B) kept at the patient's bedside and marked with the patient's name.
   (C) stored at the central nursing station.
   (D) locked in a facility safe.

6. When a patient is going to be transferred, you should make sure that the patient:

   (A) is given prior notification.
   (B) does not know about the transfer before it happens.
   (C) is fully restrained.
   (D) is being discharged.

7. During a transfer, a nursing assistant might be asked to:

   (A) ease the patient's anxiety about the move.
   (B) decide whether or not restraints are necessary.
   (C) determine what medications the patient requires.
   (D) estimate the patient's vital signs if there is no time to take them.

8. Which of the following is *not* a reason for a transfer?

   (A) A patient requests a different room
   (B) A patient's medical condition changes
   (C) A patient requires tests in another part of the facility
   (D) A patient needs assistance with toileting

9. When moving belongings during a transfer, you should:

   (A) box and label all items.
   (B) have the patient carry all of his or her belongings.
   (C) start a new patient chart and dispose of the old one.
   (D) store belongings on the stretcher or wheelchair.

10. When a patient is discharged, he or she is:

    (A) completely healed.
    (B) not expected to return to the facility.
    (C) moved to another floor or room.
    (D) recovering from surgery.

11. What does it mean when a discharge is "AMA"?

    (A) The patient is leaving before the physician thinks he or she is ready.
    (B) The patient is fully recovered.
    (C) The discharge is only temporary.
    (D) The patient is being transferred rather than discharged.

12. During a discharge, a nursing assistant might be asked to:

    (A) prescribe medication for the patient's home use.
    (B) create a new patient chart.
    (C) perform terminal cleaning of the unit.
    (D) write up discharge instructions.

_____

Signature   **Date**

The Patient's Environment

Read each statement carefully. Then circle the letter of the best answer for each item.

1. The cord or button for a call signal should always be placed:

   (A) on the wall of the patient unit.
   (B) outside the bed railing.
   (C) within the patient's reach.
   (D) in a sterile location.

2. The temperature in a patient unit should be maintained at about:

   (A) 60°F
   (B) 65°F
   (C) 70°F
   (D) 75°F

3. Windows in a patient unit should:

   (A) remain closed at all times.
   (B) provide the primary source of lighting for the room.
   (C) be blocked off with screens to block sunlight.
   (D) be opened to provide ventilation, if desirable.

4. In long-term care facilities, beds are most commonly changed:

   (A) twice a day.
   (B) daily.
   (C) once or twice a week.
   (D) once a month.

5. What is the first step in any bedmaking procedure?

   (A) Wash your hands.
   (B) Unfold the new bedding.
   (C) Remove the present bedding.
   (D) Adjust the bed to its lowest horizontal position.

6. The surgical bed is prepared for a patient who:

   (A) is returning from surgery.
   (B) is confined to the bed.
   (C) requires intravenous medication.
   (D) requires physical restraints.

7. What is the purpose of a toe pleat?

   (A) It prevents the patient's skin from touching a plastic sheet.
   (B) It reduces the pressure on the patient's feet.
   (C) It eases the transfer between the bed and the stretcher.
   (D) It prevents sheets from becoming untucked.

8. You should always wear disposable gloves when making a bed if:

   (A) the linens have been on the bed for more than one day.
   (B) the linens are soiled with blood or body fluids.
   (C) you are making a surgical bed.
   (D) you are making an occupied bed.

9. When you have finished making a closed bed, you should adjust the bed to:

   (A) its highest position.
   (B) its lowest position.
   (C) raise the head of the bed about 6 inches.
   (D) raise the foot of the bed about 6 inches.

10. A patient has been discharged from a semiprivate room. No new patient is scheduled to occupy this bed for a week. Which method of bedmaking should you use to make this bed?

    (A) Closed bed
    (B) Open bed
    (C) Occupied bed
    (D) Surgical bed

11. If a plastic draw sheet is used, you should:

    (A) rub the sheet with lotion to prevent discomfort.
    (B) use a plastic pillowcase as well.
    (C) use it as a top sheet and tuck it gently under a patient's shoulders.
    (D) completely cover it with a cotton draw sheet.

12. Glenda has been asked to change Mr. Carter's bedding. He has several greeting cards on his bed. She should:

    (A) refuse to make the bed until someone moves the cards.
    (B) tell Mr. Carter where she is placing the cards.
    (C) decide not to change the bed.
    (D) try to make the bed without moving the cards.

_____

Signature   **Date**

Hygiene and Grooming

Read each statement carefully. Then circle the letter of the best answer for each item.

1. When helping patients with their daily hygiene activities, you should encourage patients to:

   (A) do as much for themselves as possible.
   (B) bathe at least twice a day.
   (C) allow the nursing staff to take care of all hygiene needs.
   (D) limit their exercise and movements.

2. Bathing and massage can both help to stimulate:

   (A) respiration.
   (B) pulse.
   (C) circulation.
   (D) digestion.

3. When does bathing take place in most health care facilities?

   (A) As soon as patients wake up
   (B) After breakfast
   (C) After lunch
   (D) Just before going to bed

4. Most facilities consider maximum safe temperature for bath water to be:

   (A) 110°F
   (B) 130°F
   (C) 100°F
   (D) 98.6°F

5. When giving a bed bath, you should:

   (A) wash the entire body before rinsing.
   (B) wash one part of the body at a time.
   (C) never use soap.
   (D) always begin by changing the patient's bedding.

6. Most patients who are unconscious require:

   (A) little or no oral hygiene activities.
   (B) frequent mouth care.
   (C) daily bathing and shampooing.
   (D) back rubs twice a day.

7. Dentures should be washed:

   (A) about once a week.
   (B) in very hot water.
   (C) as frequently as natural teeth.
   (D) with any available disinfectant solution.

8. Which of the following tasks should *not* be performed by a nursing assistant?

   (A) Cleaning patients' hearing aids
   (B) Helping patients insert their hearing aids
   (C) Cleaning patients' eyeglasses
   (D) Checking the batteries in patients' hearing aids

9. Before trimming a patient's fingernails, you should always:

   (A) dry the nails as thoroughly as possible.
   (B) use a nail file to smooth rough edges.
   (C) give the patient a bed bath.
   (D) soak the nails in warm water.

10. When giving a patient a back rub, you should use:

    (A) disposable gloves and lotion.
    (B) warm water only.
    (C) dry hands.
    (D) plastic gloves and petroleum jelly.

11. Selma works in a long-term care facility in which residents go outside to take morning walks. She is helping Mrs. Gold with her morning activities. Selma notices that Mrs. Gold has chosen to wear a lightweight skirt although it is very cool outside. Selma should:

    (A) immediately report the problem to her supervisor.
    (B) ignore the situation to avoid embarrassing Mrs. Gold.
    (C) make Mrs. Gold aware that it is cool outside and suggest that she might be more comfortable in a different outfit.
    (D) prevent Mrs. Gold from going outside during the day.

12. Which of the following procedures is *not* recommended when shaving a male patient with a safety razor?

    (A) Using shaving cream
    (B) Holding the skin taut as you shave
    (C) Wearing disposable gloves
    (D) Using cold water to soften the beard

_____

Signature   **Date**

Special Skin Care

Read each statement carefully. Then circle the letter of the best answer for each item.

1. Which of the following does *not* describe decubitus ulcers?

   (A) Pressure sores
   (B) Fomites
   (C) Skin breakdown
   (D) Bedsores

2. Decubitus ulcers are more common in patients who are:

   (A) very active.
   (B) in rehabilitation.
   (C) on restricted diets.
   (D) elderly.

3. Decubitus ulcers are caused by:

   (A) contact with plastic sheeting.
   (B) contact with infectious materials.
   (C) prolonged pressure on the skin.
   (D) respiratory failure.

4. One common place for decubitus ulcers to appear is:

   (A) on the face.
   (B) near the tailbone.
   (C) on the neck.
   (D) on the fingers.

5. Which of the following symptoms might indicate the first stage of skin breakdown that occurs in decubitus ulcers?

   (A) A cool, dry region of skin
   (B) A lasting warm redness on the skin
   (C) A flaking of the skin similar to dandruff
   (D) An increased wrinkling or puckering of the skin

6. In which stage of skin breakdown have the layers of the skin become destroyed?

   (A) Stage one
   (B) Stage two
   (C) Stage three
   (D) Stage four

7. If skin breakdown has begun, you should:

    (A) not cover broken skin with any wrapping or bandage.
    (B) keep the area wet.
    (C) massage the affected area at least twice daily.
    (D) avoid any further pressure on the affected area.

8. Which of the following activities will *not* help to prevent decubitus ulcers?

    (A) Applying lotion to dry areas with gentle message
    (B) Making sure patients get adequate nourishment and fluids
    (C) Giving back rubs to bed-confined patients
    (D) Scrubbing skin with a rough towel to dry it

9. Which of the following conditions makes a patient more susceptible to decubitus ulcers?

    (A) Malnutrition
    (B) Stomach ulcers
    (C) Blindness
    (D) Aphasia

10. Obese patients are more likely to develop decubitus ulcers:

    (A) internally.
    (B) where body parts rub together.
    (C) around the mouth.
    (D) on the hands and feet.

11. A bed cradle is used to:

    (A) change a patient's position automatically.
    (B) redistribute a patient's weight more evenly.
    (C) prevent pressure from being concentrated in one area.
    (D) hold top linens away from the patient's skin.

12. How does sheepskin or foam padding help prevent decubitus ulcers?

    (A) It shields the skin from irritating surfaces.
    (B) It creates perspiration which lubricates the skin.
    (C) It provides important nutrients which are absorbed through the skin.
    (D) It makes a patient's skin tougher and less sensitive.

_____

Signature   **Date**

Chapter 15 • Quiz

Nutrition

Read each statement carefully. Then circle the letter of the best answer for each item.

1. Which type of nutrient provides the greatest amount of energy?

   (A) Carbohydrates
   (B) Proteins
   (C) Fats
   (D) Vitamins and minerals

2. Water does not:

   (A) aid in digestion.
   (B) regulate body temperature.
   (C) have any nutritional value.
   (D) lubricate the joints.

3. What do calories measure?

   (A) The mass or weight of a food
   (B) The energy potential of food
   (C) The nutritional value of food
   (D) The amount of water in food

4. Which of the following signs indicates poor nutrition?

   (A) Shiny-looking hair
   (B) Restful sleep patterns
   (C) Irregular elimination habits
   (D) Clear skin

5. A general diet is one that:

   (A) is a basic, well-balanced eating plan.
   (B) restricts high-calorie foods.
   (C) is prescribed by a doctor.
   (D) limits the proportions of specific foods or nutrients.

6. After surgery, the dietary routine usually begins with:

   (A) clear liquids.
   (B) soft foods.
   (C) salt-free solid foods.
   (D) dairy products.

7. You can stimulate a patient's appetite by:

(A) providing a back rub before meals.
(B) letting the patient smell the food.
(C) tasting samples of food from a patient's tray.
(D) lowering room temperature by 10°F.

8. What do the letters *NPO* indicate about a patient's diet?

(A) The patient is on a high-protein diet.
(B) The patient is on a low-fat or low-cholesterol diet.
(C) The patient should take nothing by mouth.
(D) The patient is not able to feed himself or herself.

9. Edema is a swelling of tissues that occurs when:

(A) fluid intake stops.
(B) fluid output increases.
(C) fluid output exceeds intake.
(D) fluid intake exceeds output.

10. What type of feeding provides a patient with nutrients through an opening in the abdomen?

(A) An intravenous infusion
(B) A nasogastric tube feeding
(C) A gastrostomy tube feeding
(D) A colostomy

11. Dan has been asked to monitor a patient's fluid intake. The patient has consumed only part of a carton of milk. Dan should:

(A) write down the total amount in the container.
(B) not include this fluid because the patient did not drink it all.
(C) subtract the remaining amount from the original total.
(D) immediately report the problem to his supervisor.

12. When reading the level of a fluid in a graduate, you should:

(A) hold the graduate in the air at eye level.
(B) hold the graduate at waist level.
(C) place the graduate on a bed or pillow.
(D) place the graduate on a flat surface.

Signature   **Date**

Elimination Needs

Read each statement carefully. Then circle the letter of the best answer for each item.

1. Which of the following statements about elimination frequency is true?

    (A) Most people need to urinate every 2 hours.
    (B) Most people have bowel movements once every 3 days.
    (C) Elimination frequency varies greatly from one person to another.
    (D) Elimination frequency never varies regardless of a patient's condition.

2. How frequently should you check with patients to see if they need to urinate or defecate?

    (A) Every half hour
    (B) Every 2 hours
    (C) Twice a day
    (D) Once each morning

3. You can help patients maintain normal elimination by:

    (A) restricting a patient's fluid intake.
    (B) encouraging patients to eat fiber.
    (C) discouraging exercise and activity.
    (D) stressing the importance of quickness when urinating.

4. One common cause of constipation is:

    (A) a vegetarian diet.
    (B) increased fluid intake.
    (C) exercise.
    (D) decreased fluid intake.

5. What is diarrhea?

    (A) The passage of urine through the rectum
    (B) The presence of water in a bowel movement
    (C) The passage of liquid feces
    (D) The presence of blood in a bowel movement

6. When a patient requires incontinent briefs, you should:

    (A) refer to the briefs as diapers.
    (B) wait for the patient to ask to be changed.
    (C) strictly warn the patient against bedwetting.
    (D) report any skin irritation to a supervisor.

7. A fracture pan is used by:

   (A) female patients.
   (B) male patients.
   (C) patients who cannot move easily.
   (D) patients who are incontinent.

8. When helping a patient use a bedpan in hot weather, it is a good idea to:

   (A) lubricate the seat with petroleum jelly.
   (B) dust the bedpan with powder.
   (C) place the bedpan in a refrigerator before each use.
   (D) use a metal rather than a plastic bedpan.

9. When washing the perineum, you should:

   (A) use very hot water (about 110°F).
   (B) scrub the area with a rough-textured sponge.
   (C) wash gently using a front to back stroke.
   (D) leave soap residue to protect the area.

10. A Foley catheter is used to:

    (A) help patients with chronic diarrhea.
    (B) continuously drain urine from the bladder.
    (C) decrease a patient's fluid output.
    (D) increase a patient's fluid intake.

11. The drainage bag for a catheter should be kept:

    (A) above the level of the patient's bladder.
    (B) at the same level as the patient's bladder.
    (C) below the level of the patient's bladder.
    (D) underneath the patient's leg or arm.

12. Condom catheters are:

    (A) permanently attached to the patient.
    (B) less prone to infection than Foley catheters.
    (C) replaced once or twice a month.
    (D) inserted at the urinary meatus.

_____

Signature   **Date**

Specimen Collection and Testing

Read each statement carefully. Then circle the letter of the best answer for each item.

1. A specimen is any sample of material taken from:

    (A) the lungs or bloodstream.
    (B) a patient's body.
    (C) a catheter.
    (D) microorganisms.

2. If urine samples cannot be delivered immediately, store them:

    (A) in a warm, dry location.
    (B) in a hot oven.
    (C) at room temperature.
    (D) on ice or in a refrigerator.

3. The label for a specimen should be placed:

    (A) on the lid of the container.
    (B) on the patient's chart.
    (C) in a Kardex file.
    (D) on the container itself.

4. You need to follow standard precautions:

    (A) only when collecting urine specimens.
    (B) only when collecting stool specimens.
    (C) only when collecting sputum specimens.
    (D) when collecting any specimens.

5. When collecting a midstream, clean-catch urine specimen, you should collect urine:

    (A) as soon as the urine starts to escape.
    (B) shortly after the urine starts to escape.
    (C) directly from the toilet.
    (D) for a 24-hour period.

6. Which of the following urine specimens requires two collections, 30 minutes apart?

    (A) Routine urine specimen
    (B) Midstream, clean-catch urine specimen
    (C) 24-hour urine specimen
    (D) Fresh-fractional urine specimen

7. A stool specimen is contaminated if it comes in contact with:

   (A) air.
   (B) urine.
   (C) a bedpan.
   (D) the specimen container.

8. Sputum is produced in:

   (A) the mouth.
   (B) the bloodstream.
   (C) the lungs or bronchial tubes.
   (D) the stomach.

9. Which of the following is *not* a guideline to follow when collecting a specimen?

   (A) Fill out the label carefully.
   (B) Do not touch the inside of the specimen container or lid.
   (C) Throw away unlabeled specimens.
   (D) Attach the label to the lid after you collect the specimen.

10. Specimens should never be stored:

    (A) in a refrigerator.
    (B) near food or medications.
    (C) on ice.
    (D) in plastic containers.

11. When collecting a stool specimen, you should:

    (A) try to take material from different areas of the stool.
    (B) refrigerate it if you can't take it to the lab right away.
    (C) put as much of the specimen in the container as will fit.
    (D) transport the specimen to the lab in a specimen pan.

12. Toni is collecting a routine urine specimen from a patient whose fluid intake and output is being measured. She should:

    (A) add the amount of the specimen on the I&O sheet.
    (B) subtract the amount of the specimen from the I&O sheet.
    (C) not record the procedure on the I&O sheet.
    (D) multiply the amount of the specimen by the total output.

_____

Signature   **Date**

Chapter 18 • Quiz

AM and PM Care

Read each statement carefully. Then circle the letter of the best answer for each item.

1. About how much sleep does the average adult need per night?

   (A) 3 to 5 hours
   (B) 5 to 7 hours
   (C) 7 to 9 hours
   (D) 9 to 11 hours

2. Elderly people often require:

   (A) more sleep than younger people.
   (B) less sleep than younger people.
   (C) less than 3 hours of sleep per night.
   (D) more than 9 hours of sleep per night.

3. If a person is extremely active during one day, his need for sleep that night usually:

   (A) decreases.
   (B) increases.
   (C) remains the same.
   (D) is eliminated.

4. How should you awaken a patient?

   (A) Use an alarm clock.
   (B) Place your hand on the patient's arm and say his name.
   (C) Call to the patient from outside the room.
   (D) Place a warm towel on the patient's forehead.

5. ADL such as bathing, oral hygiene, shaving, hair care, and dressing are usually performed:

   (A) before breakfast.
   (B) after breakfast.
   (C) after lunch.
   (D) before sleep.

6. What is HS care?

   (A) Bedtime care
   (B) Assistance conducting the activities of daily living
   (C) Preparation for a transfer
   (D) Helping the patient turn in bed

7. Which of the following activities is especially helpful for promoting sleep?

   (A) A back rub
   (B) Exercise
   (C) Taking a patient's vital signs
   (D) Positioning the patient in the Fowler's position

8. Older patients are more likely than younger patients to:

   (A) sleep heavily without waking.
   (B) sleep for more than 10 hours.
   (C) have difficulty falling back to sleep after awakening.
   (D) awake fully rested.

9. Which of the following activities is not usually considered a routine part of AM care?

   (A) Waking the patient
   (B) Assisting with toileting
   (C) Giving the patient the opportunity to brush teeth and wash face and hands
   (D) Preparing a patient for surgery

10. Ms. Gould has surgery in the morning so she cannot eat breakfast. The nursing assistant should:

    (A) wake Ms. Gould as early as possible.
    (B) wake Ms. Gould at least 5 hours before surgery.
    (C) allow Ms. Gould to sleep through breakfast time.
    (D) prescribe sleeping pills to help Ms. Gould sleep.

11. Mr. Martinez prefers to shower before breakfast, even though it is more common for patients in his facility to shower after breakfast. The nursing assistant should:

    (A) allow Mr. Martinez to make his preference part of the routine.
    (B) insist that Mr. Martinez shower after breakfast.
    (C) allow Mr. Martinez to choose his preference, but refuse to help.
    (D) report the problem immediately to the supervisor.

12. When providing PM care, a nursing assistant should always:

    (A) leave the overbed light on throughout the night.
    (B) put fresh drinking water within the patient's reach.
    (C) make sure that the patient does not eat any snacks.
    (D) turn on a television or radio softly.

_____

Signature   **Date**

124

Restorative Care and Rehabilitation

Read each statement carefully. Then circle the letter of the best answer for each item.

1. The goal of rehabilitation is to help patients:

    (A) maintain a level of health and well-being.
    (B) regain the highest possible state of functioning.
    (C) reduce the length of their stay in a health care facility.
    (D) create a complete treatment plan.

2. Which member of the interdisciplinary team teaches patients how to take an active part in the tasks of daily care?

    (A) Psychologist
    (B) Physical therapist
    (C) Speech therapist
    (D) Occupational therapist

3. Which of the following is an assistive device?

    (A) A food guard
    (B) The call signal
    (C) The patient's chart
    (D) A dietary supplement

4. A prosthesis is:

    (A) an activity of daily living.
    (B) a device used to cushion the patient in bed.
    (C) a device used to support a part of the body.
    (D) an artificial body part.

5. Back braces and knee immobilizers are examples of:

    (A) prostheses.
    (B) diseases.
    (C) orthotics.
    (D) medications.

6. To help with bladder retraining, you should:

    (A) scold the patient for unnecessary incontinence.
    (B) discourage fluid intake.
    (C) never run water in the sink to prompt urination.
    (D) offer the patient the opportunity to toilet at the prescribed times.

7. A patient with total incontinence has a complete lack of:

   (A) ambulation.
   (B) bowel or bladder control.
   (C) blood pressure.
   (D) mobility.

8. How long does it usually take to retrain incontinent patients?

   (A) 2 to 4 days
   (B) 5 to 12 days
   (C) 2 to 3 weeks
   (D) 6 to 10 weeks

9. Because it is a time at which most people feel the urge to defecate, you should encourage patients to toilet:

   (A) before going to sleep.
   (B) before breakfast.
   (C) after breakfast.
   (D) after exercise.

10. What is spasticity?

    (A) Hyperactive behavior
    (B) A muscle's continuous resistance to stretching
    (C) Damage to muscles caused by range-of-motion exercises
    (D) The ability to move limbs through their full range of motion

11. When carrying out passive range-of-motion exercises, you should use:

    (A) sharp, strong movements.
    (B) as much force as you can.
    (C) slow, gentle movements.
    (D) enough force to push a joint slightly past its point of resistance.

12. If the arm or leg is moved away from the center of the body, the exercise is called:

    (A) dorsal flexion.
    (B) plantar flexion.
    (C) abduction.
    (D) supination.

_____

Signature   **Date**

126

Chapter 20 • Quiz

Additional Patient Care Procedures

Read each statement carefully. Then circle the letter of the best answer for each item.

1. Heat treatments are used to:

    (A) dilate blood vessels.
    (B) increase pulse.
    (C) constrict blood vessels.
    (D) decrease pulse.

2. How can you tell if a patient has cyanosis?

    (A) Skin appears blue
    (B) Hair falls out
    (C) Teeth chatter
    (D) Lips become dry and chapped

3. Which of the following is not a safety guideline to follow when applying a cold treatment?

    (A) Place a cloth cover or towel around the pack, pad, or bag.
    (B) Apply the pack or pad directly to the patient's skin.
    (C) Make sure metal lids on ice caps face away from the skin.
    (D) Check the skin frequently for signs of complication.

4. Which of the following is a dry heat treatment?

    (A) Heat lamp
    (B) Sitz bath
    (C) Cleansing enema
    (D) Oil-retention enema

5. Cold compresses are left in place no longer than:

    (A) 2 minutes.
    (B) 20 minutes.
    (C) 1 hour.
    (D) 3 hours.

6. Which of the following treatments can be applied only by a licensed nurse?

    (A) A sterile compress
    (B) A sponge bath
    (C) A cold soak
    (D) A sitz bath

7. An aquamatic pad is used to provide:

   (A) dry heat treatment.
   (B) moist heat treatment.
   (C) dry cold treatment.
   (D) moist cold treatment.

8. Which of the following instruments is used to examine the ears?

   (A) Sphygmomanometer
   (B) Emesis basin
   (C) Otoscope
   (D) Ophthalmoscope

9. A nasal speculum is used to examine:

   (A) reflexes.
   (B) the nose.
   (C) the eyes.
   (D) the pulse.

10. The purpose of a cleansing enema is to:

    (A) relieve constipation.
    (B) eliminate incontinence.
    (C) relieve abdominal distention.
    (D) remove feces from the rectum and colon.

11. Before administering an enema, the patient should be in the:

    (A) semi-Fowler's position.
    (B) prone position.
    (C) left-lying Sims' position.
    (D) reverse Trendelenburg position.

12. Which of the following activities is *not* recommended when administering an enema?

    (A) Allowing the patient to use the bathroom before the procedure
    (B) Giving the enema before the patient's bath
    (C) Inserting the tubing only 3 inches into the rectum
    (D) Administering the solution as quickly as possible

13. Which of the following is the correct amount of time to leave a rectal tube in place?

    (A) 3 hours
    (B) 6 hours
    (C) 20 minutes once a day
    (D) 20 minutes three times a day

_____

Signature   **Date**

Preoperative and Postoperative Care

Read each statement carefully. Then circle the letter of the best answer for each item.

1. A patient should be prepared and ready:

   (A) 10 minutes before the scheduled time of surgery.
   (B) 1 hour before the time of surgery.
   (C) 4 hours before the time of surgery.
   (D) the night before surgery.

2. When transporting a patient to the operating room on a stretcher, you should:

   (A) make sure the straps are unbuckled.
   (B) push the stretcher slowly.
   (C) remove all sheets and blankets from the stretcher.
   (D) place the patient's personal belongings under the stretcher.

3. Removing a patient's hair at the surgical site may be done before surgery to prevent:

   (A) cancer.
   (B) contamination.
   (C) allergies.
   (D) signs of aging.

4. What is a depilatory?

   (A) A cream used for hair removal
   (B) A tool used to remove stitches
   (C) A restraining device used on stretchers
   (D) A disinfectant used to prevent bacterial growth

5. A local anesthesia blocks the reception of pain:

   (A) throughout the body.
   (B) in the brain only.
   (C) only in the area to be operated on.
   (D) in the limbs.

6. A spinal anesthetic usually causes loss of feeling:

   (A) in the arms.
   (B) from the navel down to the feet.
   (C) along the spinal column.
   (D) in the head and neck.

7. When vomited materials are aspirated, they are:

   (A) expelled through the mouth.
   (B) expelled through the nose.
   (C) drawn back into the stomach.
   (D) drawn back into the lungs.

8. Only a physician or a nurse can:

   (A) observe a patient's vital signs after an operation.
   (B) report signs of leakage from intravenous lines.
   (C) adjust the rate of infusion of the IV solution.
   (D) check for obstructions in the urinary drainage system.

9. Which of the following is *not* a part of routine postoperative care?

   (A) Skin preparation
   (B) Range-of-motion exercises for the legs
   (C) Deep-breathing exercises
   (D) Binders and stockings

10. Deep-breathing exercises help to prevent:

    (A) cardiovascular disease.
    (B) pneumonia.
    (C) rehabilitation.
    (D) circulation.

11. What type of binders are used to hold dressings in the anal area in place?

    (A) Scultetus binders
    (B) Abdominal binders
    (C) Elasticized stockings
    (D) T-binders

12. Which of the following activities helps a patient to prepare for ambulation?

    (A) Sleeping
    (B) Dangling
    (C) Coughing
    (D) Shaving

_____

Signature   **Date**

Subacute Care

Read each statement carefully. Then circle the letter of the best answer for each item.

1. Subacute care can best be described as:

   (A) improvisational care.
   (B) substandard care.
   (C) transformational care.
   (D) transitional care.

2. The nursing assistant who works in a subacute care facility is often called a:

   (A) PGA.
   (B) ATA.
   (C) TTT or ITT.
   (D) TCA or CENA.

3. Compared with hospital care, subacute care is _____ expensive.

   (A) equally
   (B) more
   (C) less
   (D) much more

4. Subacute care patients are classified according to their potential to _____ with care.

   (A) improve
   (B) disapprove
   (C) regress
   (D) approve

5. When working on a team, it is important to understand your own _____ as well as that of the other team members.

   (A) fate
   (B) well-being
   (C) role
   (D) salary

6. The environment in subacute care units or facilities can be very:

   (A) confusing.
   (B) noisy.
   (C) boring.
   (D) complex.

7. If a patient vomits while a stomach tube is in place, you should:

   (A) remove the tube immediately.
   (B) notify the nurse immediately.
   (C) go to lunch.
   (D) clean up the mess.

8. A wound that becomes contaminated with feces might get:

   (A) infected.
   (B) rejected.
   (C) noticed.
   (D) better.

9. To get paid by the insurance companies, the subacute facility's care of the patient must match:

   (A) the prescribed treatment plan.
   (B) for all patients.
   (C) hospital care.
   (D) at all times.

10. When the goals of the care plan are met, the patient:

   (A) is cured.
   (B) always goes home.
   (C) is readmitted to the hospital.
   (D) may go home or to a long-term care facility.

_____

Signature   **Date**

Chapter 23 • Quiz

Special Skills in Long-Term Care

Read each statement carefully. Then circle the letter of the best answer for each item.

1. The majority of residents in nursing homes are:

   (A) elderly.
   (B) disabled.
   (C) men.
   (D) infants.

2. When people move into a nursing home, expect them to:

   (A) adjust in a day or two.
   (B) need time to adjust.
   (C) no longer have any contact with family.
   (D) no longer have sexual needs.

3. Which of the following activities is *not* an example of age-appropriate behavior for an 80-year-old man?

   (A) Playing poker
   (B) Reading books
   (C) Solving crossword puzzles
   (D) Starting a food fight

4. Whenever possible, you should try to:

   (A) discourage family members from visiting a nursing home.
   (B) discourage residents from using the telephone.
   (C) prepare residents for visitors.
   (D) prevent family members from helping to provide daily care.

5. Masturbation is:

   (A) physically harmful to the elderly.
   (B) emotionally harmful to the elderly.
   (C) acceptable behavior for satisfying sexual needs.
   (D) always appropriate, regardless of the situation.

6. Which of the following activities can help to satisfy an individual's spiritual needs?

   (A) Gardening
   (B) Attending a church service
   (C) Making handicrafts
   (D) Conducting activities of daily living

7. As people age, their sense of taste:

    (A) diminishes.
    (B) increases.
    (C) is completely lost.
    (D) affects their balance.

8. Compared to those of a young woman, an older woman's bones are:

    (A) more brittle and porous.
    (B) harder and stronger.
    (C) softer and more flexible.
    (D) more sensitive to pain.

9. The general term given to symptoms associated with the chronic, organic decline of mental ability is:

    (A) dementia.
    (B) Alzheimer's disease.
    (C) paranoia.
    (D) depression.

10. Which of the following factors is *not* one of the most common triggers of difficult behavior in cognitively impaired people?

    (A) Fatigue
    (B) Too much stimulation
    (C) Relaxation
    (D) Change of routine or environment

11. Which of the following questions is best suited for a resident with dementia?

    (A) "What do you want for lunch today?"
    (B) "Would you rather have peas or carrots?"
    (C) "Where would you like to eat lunch today?"
    (D) "How many different foods would you like for lunch today?"

12. What can you do to lessen the problems caused by sundowning?

    (A) Avoid scheduling activities late in the day.
    (B) Provide the resident with a "rummaging" box.
    (C) Vary the resident's daily routine.
    (D) Exercise the resident late in the day.

_____

Signature   **Date**

Death and Dying

Read each statement carefully. Then circle the letter of the best answer for each item.

1. A terminal illness is an illness or injury:

   (A) inherited from the parents.
   (B) caused by contact with a health care facility.
   (C) from which the patient will not recover.
   (D) that affects the respiratory system.

2. According to Dr. Kübler-Ross, the first stage of emotional experience in terminally ill people in facing their illness is:

   (A) depression.
   (B) denial.
   (C) anger.
   (D) acceptance.

3. A terminally ill patient says she plans to live long enough to see the birth of her first grandchild due in 6 months. This illustrates:

   (A) denial.
   (B) acceptance.
   (C) bargaining.
   (D) anger.

4. Attitudes about death:

   (A) are the same in every culture.
   (B) do not vary as a person ages.
   (C) are influenced by religion.
   (D) need not be identified by a nursing assistant.

5. Before assuming the care of dying patients, it is important that you:

   (A) understand your own feelings about death.
   (B) have experienced the death of a loved one.
   (C) have gone through the five stages of emotional experience.
   (D) learn about medications that help ease pain.

6. During the dying process, a patient's vision becomes:

(A) sensitive to bright colors.
(B) sensitive to darkness.
(C) blurred and gradually fails.
(D) vivid and precise.

7. One of the last functions to be lost is the sense of:

(A) hearing.
(B) sight.
(C) taste.
(D) smell.

8. The mouths of terminally ill patients often become:

(A) overly moist.
(B) dry.
(C) swollen.
(D) blue or purple.

9. During a Catholic patient's confession, you must:

(A) remain as quiet as possible.
(B) sit beside the patient to observe vital signs.
(C) leave the room.
(D) prevent the priest from touching the patient.

10. What does a *DNR* or "*no code*" notation on a patient's record mean?

(A) Efforts should not be made to resuscitate the patient.
(B) No food is to be taken orally.
(C) The patient has refused all medication.
(D) The patient is terminally ill.

11. Which of the following changes does *not* occur after death?

(A) Pupils become fixed and dilated.
(B) Body heat increases.
(C) Urine, feces, and flatus are released.
(D) Rigor mortis occurs.

12. A hospital's holding area for bodies is called:

(A) a cemetery.
(B) an autopsy.
(C) a postmortem.
(D) a morgue.

_____

Signature   **Date**